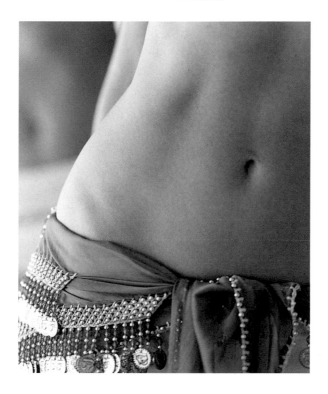

bellydance

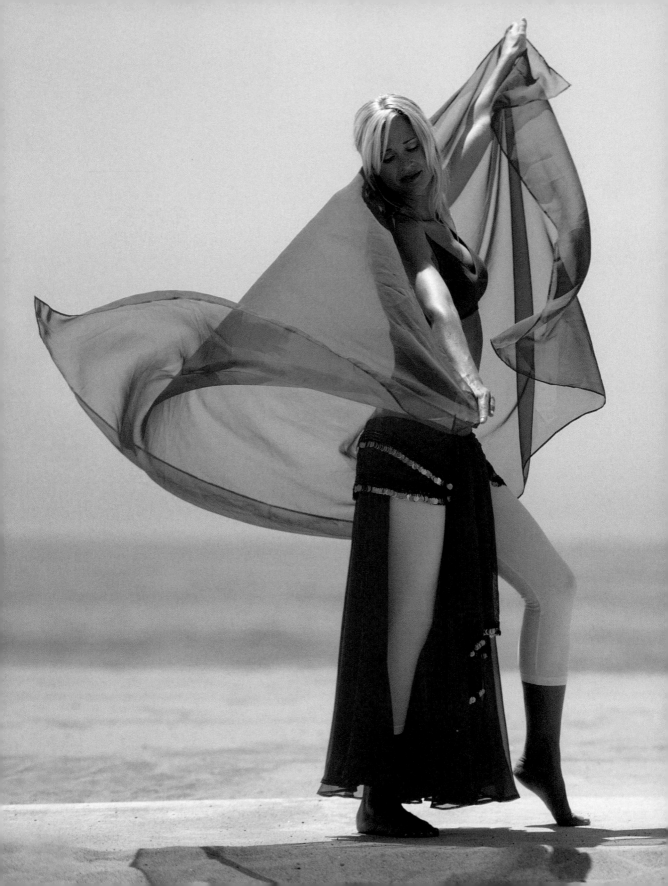

bellydance

Dolphina

Photography by

John Robbins

DK Publishing, Inc.

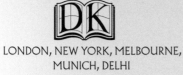

LONDON, NEW YORK, MELBOURNE,
MUNICH, DELHI

For all women

Project Editor   Nasim Mawji
Art Editor   Susan St. Louis
Assistant Managing Art Editor   Michelle Baxter
Additional Design   Miesha Tate, Melissa Chung,
Jessica Lasher, Tai Blanche, Belinda Hock
DTP Coordinator   Milos Orlovic
Production Manager   Chris Avgherinos
Jacket Design   Dirk Kaufman
Project Director   Sharon Lucas
Creative Director   Tina Vaughan

Photography   John Robbins
Photographic Assistants   Troy Bass, Alex de Groot

First American Edition 2005
04 05 06 07 10 9 8 7 6 5 4 3 2 1

Published in the United States by
DK Publishing, Inc.
375 Hudson Street
New York, New York 10014

Always consult your doctor before starting a fitness
program if you have any concerns.

DK Publishing offers special discounts for bulk purchases for sales
promotions of premiums. Specific, large-quanity needs can be
met with special editions, including personalized covers,
excerpts of existing guides, and corporate imprints.
For more information, contact:
Special Markets Department
DK Publishing, Inc.
375 Hudson Street
New York, New York 10014
Fax: 212-689-5254

Cataloging-in-Publication data is available
from the Library of Congress.
ISBN: 0-7566-0555-5

Color reproduction by GRB Editrice, srl, Italy
Printed and bound in Singapore by Tien Wah Press Pte Ltd.

See our complete product line at
www.dk.com

CONTENTS

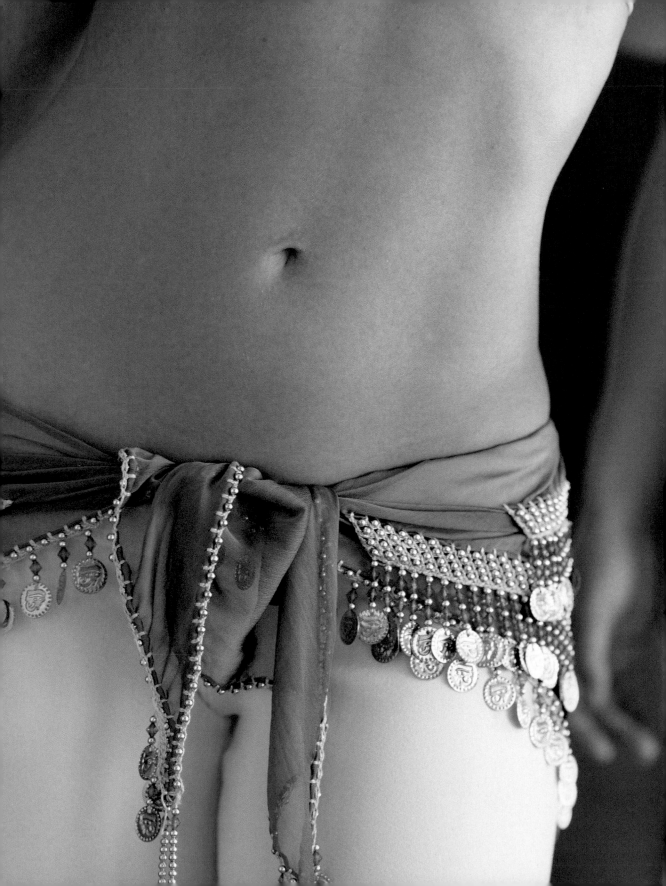

WHAT IS BELLY DANCE?

If you have ever watched a bellydancer,
you have probably been held mesmerized by
her hypnotic movements. Each shimmy and
graceful undulation is an expression of strength
and femininity. This book introduces you to all
the essential elements of bellydance. It shows you
how this ancient art form can not only provide
an exhilarating workout that increases flexibility
and tones your entire body, it can boost
your confidence and empower you.

DEFINING BELLYDANCE

Bellydance is perhaps the oldest form of dance. Its origins can be traced back to ancient Oriental, Indian, and Middle Eastern cultures. Although many people today think of it as a seductive dance intended to entertain men, in fact men have only been permitted to observe this unique art form in its more recent history. Traditionally bellydance was performed by women for women as part of ancient fertility rituals and goddess worship ceremonies.

In Arabic, bellydance is known as *raks sharqi*, which literally translates as "dance from the East;" you may also see it referred to as *danse Orientale*. There are several different theories on how it came to be known as bellydance in the West. It is similar in sound to the Arabic name for "dance of the people," or *beledi*, but a more likely explanation is that it came from the French "*danse du ventre*," or "dance of the stomach."

THE ORIGINS

Because bellydance spans so many cultures, its exact origins are difficult to pinpoint. What I find fascinating is its connection with fertility rituals practiced in the Stone Age. Many ancient artifacts depicting women as deities exist (far more than images of men), which has led archaeologists to speculate that women were dominant and considered sacred in Stone Age society. Women would have danced together to honor Mother Earth in spiritual ceremonies and were taught to dance as a way to celebrate and worship their goddess, for sexual fertility, and in preparation for childbirth. It seems likely that this ritualistic dancing formed the

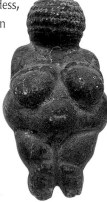

The Venus of Willendorf, one of humankind's oldest recorded pieces of art. This small stone sculpture dates back some 25, 000 years and is believed by many archaeologists to be evidence of ancient matriarchal societies.

foundations of modern bellydance as we know it today. The undulating movements and its focus on the hips, abdominals, and chest suggest a connection to female fertility, in both conception and labor.

THE HISTORY

The legacy of women bellydancing for women continued well into the more recent history of bellydance. In the harems of Constantinople in the mid-1400s, female gypsy bellydancers were hired to entertain the women, not the Sultan. They danced the Turkish style of bellydance, with finger cymbals and earthy movements performed on the floor.

Some gypsy tribes traveled to Egypt and developed the very popular, *ghawazee* folk-style of dance that incorporated many showy props such as veils, candles, and swords that are still used today. By the beginning of the nineteenth century men were catching their first glimpses of bellydance, since *ghawazee* dancing was being performed outside in makeshift theaters where the gypsies laid their carpets. In 1834, Cairo's religious restrictions forced bellydance underground, although it re-emerged in the 1850s.

As Europeans began to travel more, their fascination with North Africa and the Middle East began to grow. Artists such as Renoir, Matisse, and Ingres all painted harem women, and in 1893 Oscar Wilde staged *Salome* in London, which featured the seductive "Dance of the Seven Veils." A cultural phenomenon known as "Salomania" began to spread through Europe.

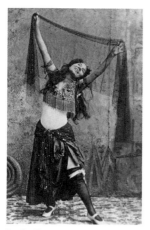

Little Egypt gave Americans their first taste of bellydance.

Salomania reached America in 1893 when a dancer named Little Egypt (thought to be Algerian) performed at the Chicago World's Fair. Her exotic movements were considered outrageous for the times, but audiences were entranced, and bellydancers made apearances in many of Hollywood's early silent films.

By the turn of the century nightclubs were beginning to open in North Africa and the Middle East to meet the demands of the colonial rulers and Western tourists. Audiences paid to watch glamorous bellydancers dressed in ornate costumes. They danced on their toes, performing subtle hip movements and graceful arm and hand gestures, very like modern Egyptian-style bellydance.

Before being accused of being a German spy during World War One, Mata Hari was renowned in Europe for her exotic dance routines. Society's attitudes were changing, and exotic dancing was becoming a form of liberation and glamorous empowerment for women.

Bellydance influences reached far and wide and even inspired the greats of modern dance, including Isadora Duncan, Ruth St. Denis, and Martha Graham.

During the Women's Liberation movement of the 1970s bellydance experienced another revival. This was largely due to the release of an album by a Turkish bellydancer, Ozel Turkbas, which also included an instructional booklet on how to bellydance. During the sexual revolution, bellydance was embraced by a generation of women who were captivated by the liberating movements, belly-exposing costumes, and camaraderie with other women. Classes sprung up at YWCAs across America, "hip-huggers" and "bikinis" celebrated women's bare bellies for the first time in fashion history, and bellydance was featured in

Life magazine. As the dance gained in popularity, it became a way for women everywhere to affirm their individual magnificence and power.

Today, bellydance is more popular than ever as women begin to realize its fitness potential. Many women now enjoy an ancient dance as their regular form of exercise. Past and present, bellydance encourages each woman to celebrate her personal inner beauty.

The most astonishing and beautiful aspect of bellydance's colorful and rich history is that the dance not only endured but also evolved and adapted to suit the current social and political situation. To this day it continues its legacy as a source of female empowerment.

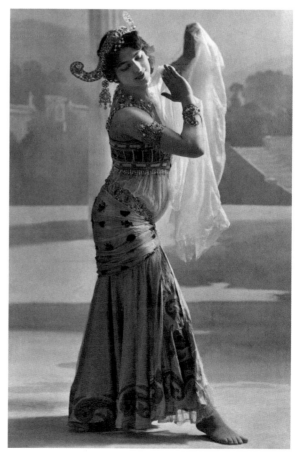

Considered scandalous by many, Mata Hari performed "Oriental style" exotic dances with veils and shawls. Her provocative routines aroused intense public interest.

WHY BELLYDANCE?

Bellydance is a total workout for the body, mind, and spirit. Not only does it provide a thorough, non-impact, and fat-burning exercise that tones and sculpts your muscles, it actually promotes a positive mental attitude about your body. Women who bellydance feel more confident and at ease with their figures—and you don't need to be slim to begin bellydancing. Goddesses come in all shapes and sizes.

THE BENEFITS

One of the most powerful benefits of bellydance can be experienced the very first time you make a simple Figure Eight with your hips. The act of gyrating your abdominals, buns, and thighs (parts of the body associated with femininity) in new and pleasurable ways, rather than in squats and crunches, causes a liberating shift in attitude. After bellydancing, don't be surprised to find yourself bursting with newfound confidence.

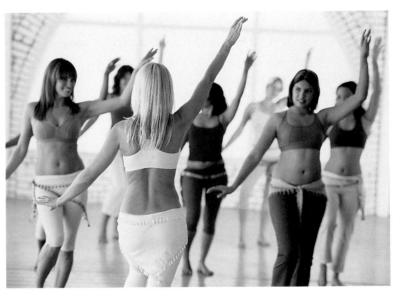

Try taking a bellydance class; women from all walks of life enjoy bellydance as a fun and liberating form of exercise.

The numerous physical benefits of bellydance make it an ideal stand-alone workout, or you can practice it to enhance your existing fitness regimen. It is an excellent cardiovascular exercise that also improves flexibility and muscle tone. Most women have concerns about their abdominals, buns, and thighs, and these muscles can be effectively sculpted with regular bellydance. Unlike any other exercise, bellydance isolates specific muscle groups. As you move one set, you hold other muscle groups completely still. This dynamic lengthens your muscles, eventually toning and strengthening them. For example, holding your chest still while your hips move in serpentine Figure Eights, sculpts the muscles at the sides of the torso (your obliques) and defines the waist.

Because much of the movement is generated from the torso rather than the arms and legs, bellydance is also very effective at building "core" strength. It works the muscles in the upper body, abdominals, and pelvic area, which can help promote good posture. Apart from stimulating circulation and improving coordination, an hour-long bellydance session provides a feeling of freedom and release that will be a totally new and revitalizing experience for many.

Women today lead busy and hectic lives, but a bellydance session provides an opportunity to claim time for yourself and escape from the mundane. You'll find that performing these intensely feminine movements helps you leave behind the stresses and strains of modern day life and reawaken the woman within.

THE GODDESS WORKOUT

Bellydance has always been an important part of my life. I first began learning from my mother at the age of four when she took me with her to her bellydance classes. I lived in Morocco as a child, and I remember being mesmerized by bellydancers who moved with such grace and control and seemed effortlessly able to ripple one stomach muscle at a time. These early experiences inspired me to study dance later in life. I practiced many different styles, but was always influenced by the graceful and rhythmic movements of bellydance. I stayed in shape predominantly by bellydancing, but also by supplementing my exercise regimen with yoga and Pilates classes. I realised that there was a real fascination with bellydance— women continuously asked me about it and wanted to learn how to do it. It wasn't until I qualified as a fitness instructor that I felt ready to devise a workout based on my own exercise routine. I broke down the basic bellydance moves and incorporated stretching, muscle toning, and aerobic elements to create the Goddess Workout—so called because I wanted to convey the empowering feelings that bellydancing arouse in me.

Through bellydance I discovered my Goddess within. It has been my form of fitness, my meditation, my creativity, my entertainment, and my way of life. When I am bellydancing, layers of self-doubt fall away to reveal a confident woman.

I have discovered a secret through bellydance—one that I intend to share with you in this book. I hope that bellydance can be as great a source of inspiration for you as it has been for me, and that you find it an effective and, most importantly, enjoyable way to get— and stay—in shape.

KEEPING MOTIVATED

Following any fitness regimen requires a certain degree of commitment and motivation, no matter how pleasurable the exercise. Try these tips for keeping you on track:

1. Schedule workouts Make it difficult to cancel by arranging to work out with a friend or by taking a private bellydance class. Commit, or you will never find that "extra time" to work out.

2. Dress up Wear a coin- or bead-fringed hip scarf when you work out. Accessories improve technique and make bellydancing feel less like exercise.

3. Make it fun Learn more about traditional bellydance music (see pp150–151), or throw a bellydance party (see pp152–153).

4. Have the right attitude This is your time—treat it as your opportunity to take care of your feminine spirit.

5. Be inspired Post photographs of women you admire (I call them goddesses), in places where you may need inspiration or resolve, such as your closet or the door of your refrigerator.

6. Set goals Achieving goals will motivate you. Begin small: Say, "I will do 10 figure eights." Then do them.

7. Reward yourself Buy yourself small gifts such as new music or bellydance accessories when you achieve your workout goals.

8. Obey the five-minute rule Commit to working out for at least five minutes at a time. Stop if you feel tired after five minutes, but you probably won't want to. The hurdle is always getting started.

9. Don't overdo it Start slowly, and listen to your body. As your fitness level improves, extend the length of your workout period and exercise more often. You will avoid injury and burnout by building your fitness level slowly.

10. Sign up for a class Commit to a series of regular bellydance classes. You will meet people, get involved in the scene, and make friends.

MOVEMENT PRINCIPLES

When you bellydance, you'll discover muscles that you didn't know existed and learn to use them in new and unusual ways. Understanding the basic movement principles is essential, since they not only provide the foundations for good technique, they will prevent you from putting unnecessary strain on the body. Keep these principles in mind and you'll notice how you begin to feel more at ease with and aware of your body as you learn the shimmies, shakes, and flowing, sensual movements of bellydance.

MUSCLE ISOLATION

This is the most fundamental movement principle. As you move one set of muscles, you hold the other muscle groups still. This technique not only intensively works specific muscles, strengthening and toning them, it helps to draw attention to the moving part of the body. For example, holding your chest still while you perform Figure Eights emphasizes the serpentine movements of your hips. It may be difficult to master this at first, but it won't take long for your upper abdominal muscles to become accustomed to being targeted in this way. You may not be able to keep your chest perfectly still when you initially practice the Figure Eight, but it will help you to focus the movement on your upper abdominal muscles. Each time you practice a move, you will notice how your ability to isolate specific muscle groups improves.

MUSCLE CONTROL

There may be muscles that you regularly use in other forms of exercise that suddenly burn when you begin bellydancing. This is because you are using the muscle in a different way. For example, you might be strong in your triceps and biceps from lifting weights, but it is quite possible that your arms will tire easily when practicing the undulating movements of Snake Arms.

Muscle control is essential for creating both the smooth, fluid movements and the sharp, dramatic ones that are so characteristic of bellydance. Sometimes the movements will require you to move your muscles in unusual ways. For example, when performing a Hip Camel, you push out your abdominal muscles, which may feel awkward at first (especially if you are used to contracting your abdominals to keep your tummy tucked in).

The muscles you use and the way in which you work them in bellydance will also be different to other forms of exercise. People generally aren't familiar with the iliopsoas, a muscle that runs from the lower back to the thighbone and is important for good posture and hip mobility. It is common for this muscle to be tight if you have a sedentary job, yet it is rarely targeted in ordinary gym exercise. However it is used often when performing hip movements in bellydance.

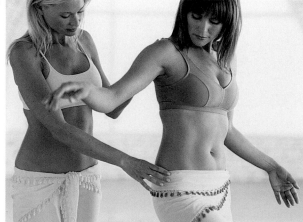

Be aware of your body as you practice new moves, and you'll notice how you start to feel muscles that you may not have used before.

BALANCE AND FLOW

Many of the movements in bellydance focus on the hips. A key point to remember is that all hip movements are generated by bending the knees as you shift your weight. Distributing your weight correctly helps your balance and coordination. It also allows you more control over the pace of your movements—so that they appear sharp or soft but always retain a mesmerizing flow. Finally, I'll remind you throughout the book to keep your knees slightly bent, or "soft," when performing a move or even when standing in the Basic Stance (*see pp16–17*). Locking your knees straight can make your movements appear jerky.

EXPRESSION

Dance is a form of expression. Although good technique is important when learning to bellydance, it is just as important to discover the joy and freedom that comes from moving your body in pleasurable ways. The movements of bellydance celebrate the feminine form and should feel natural to perform. Practice and learn the Basic Moves, but when you perform them as part of a dance, allow yourself to experience the liberating feeling that comes from "letting go." This wonderful sensation will stay with you even after your workout is over—and you may find that it adds excitement to other areas of your life too!

MUSCLE STRUCTURE

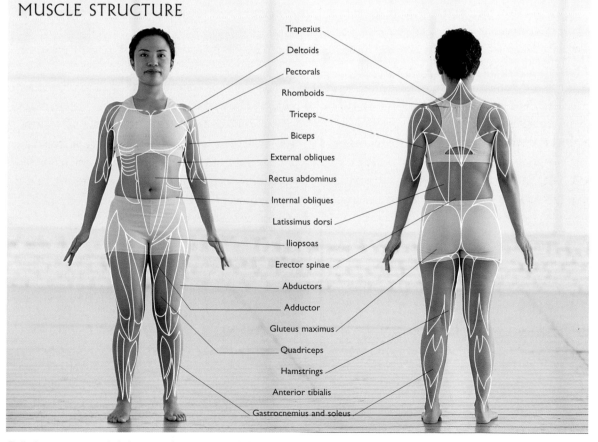

Trapezius
Deltoids
Pectorals
Rhomboids
Triceps
Biceps
External obliques
Rectus abdominus
Internal obliques
Latissimus dorsi
Iliopsoas
Erector spinae
Abductors
Adductor
Gluteus maximus
Quadriceps
Hamstrings
Anterior tibialis
Gastrocnemius and soleus

Bellydance tones and defines nearly every muscle in the body, but the most visible results occur in the abdominal region. Bellydance sculpts the entire stomach because it targets the internal and external obliques (the side abdominals) as well as the entire rectus abdominus (the upper and lower abdominals).

GETTING STARTED

Taking your first steps as a bellydancer couldn't be simpler—you don't need special clothing, and even music is not essential (although it can help you to keep a steady rhythm). Here I offer some basic guidelines for getting started that will not only increase your enjoyment of bellydance, but will help you benefit physically from it.

HOW TO USE THIS BOOK

The purpose of this book is to provide step-by-step instruction on how to bellydance for fun and fitness. It will be as useful to the novice as to the experienced bellydancer who simply wants to perfect her technique.

The basic moves are presented in three levels, each one progressing in difficulty. At the end of each basic moves section, a three-part choreographed routine provides you with a suggested sequence that links the basic moves learned in that section to form a dance.

There are several ways to use this book, depending on your desired goals. I recommend warming up with the Goddess Salutation, my simple stretching routine. Then the novice bellydancer should begin with Basic Moves Level One. Practice each move slowly, learning the breakdowns and focusing on the muscle isolations.

The Tips and Technique box that accompanies each move tells you where you should feel a move when you are isolating the right muscles and performing it correctly. Once you have learned the moves in level one, go on to the corresponding dance routine. Work your way through the book, progressing to the next level when you feel ready.

You can also use this book to target specific muscles, with the aim of toning and sculpting them. In this case, follow the recommended Workout Repetitions for each move. If you are new to bellydance or do not exercise regularly, follow the guidelines for the Beginner level and aim to workout two to three times a week for between 30 and 45 minutes at a time. Otherwise, follow the Intermediate level, working out with the same frequency.

WHAT TO WEAR

Although professional bellydancers often wear elaborate costumes, wear anything that allows you to move freely when you first begin learning. I recommend leggings and a tank-top or t-shirt. You do not need to expose your belly. Eventually, however, you will want to see the movements you are making by wearing a bra top or a midriff top. If you are just beginning, tie a scarf or shawl around your hips, since this immediately makes you more aware of them as you move. You could invest in a hip scarf, preferably a coin- or bead-fringed one because it will help you to hear the rhythm of your movements. (See page 156 for advice on where to buy hip scarves.)

Bellydance is a no-impact exercise, so you do not need to wear shoes, and in fact it is traditional to dance barefoot, since this affirms your connection with the earth and will enhance your feelings of liberation. Ultimately, I encourage you to wear an outfit that makes you feel beautiful, chic, strong, sexy, and glamorous. This will help you to enjoy your bellydance session and make it feel less like a workout. You may discover that you develop a real interest in bellydance costumes and accessories— certainly part of the appeal for many people.

For the routines in this book, the costumes consist of a bra top, leggings, and a hip scarf. In the Goddess Dance (see pp94–109) and Veil Dance (see pp130–145), the dancers tied a hip scarf over a simple chiffon skirt made up of an elastic waist and two panels of chiffon, one at the back, one at the front.

Wear comfortable clothing that won't restrict your movements, and enjoy dancing barefoot.

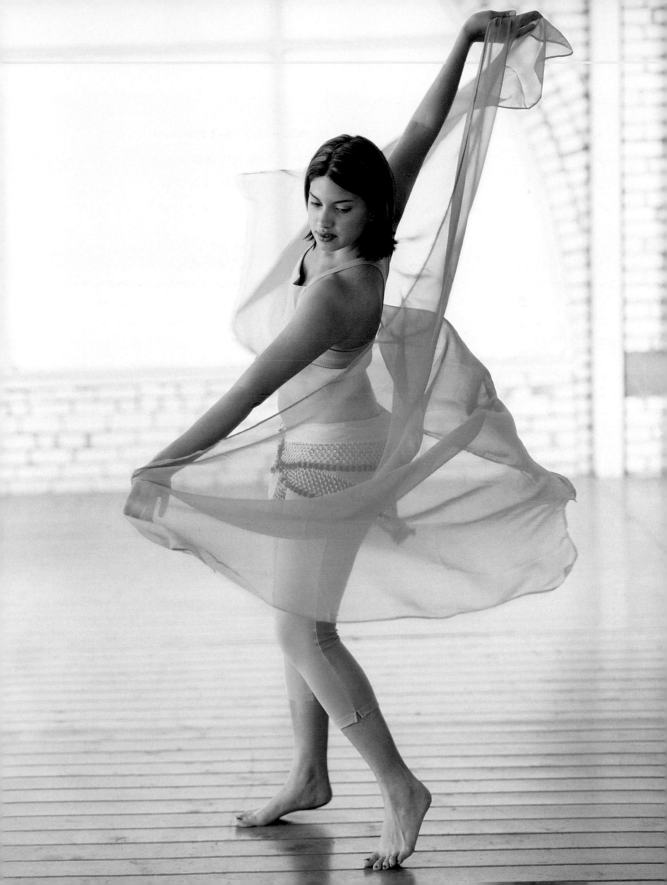

MUSIC AND RHYTHM

Whether it's traditional Moroccan drums, heavy metal, or The Beatles, the music you play during your bellydance practice should inspire you to dance. Dance is a visual expression of music; therefore, you need to learn to count in musical terms. Those new to bellydancing or unfamiliar with Middle Eastern music, will probably find it easier to learn to count to Western music, since it usually has a regular 4/4 rhythm. For more information on Middle Eastern music, including classic bellydance songs, see pages 150–151. See page 155 for advice on where to shop for music.

For now, try this simple exercise to help you learn how to count the beats in music: Choose two songs, one fast and upbeat for the sharp moves, and one slow and sensual for the fluid and slow moves. Listen to the music and begin counting to eight; repeat until you have found the rhythm and can count a regular beat. When you learn the basic moves, you can count each step which will help your rhythm as well as your coordination. Being aware of the rhythm will also help you to link the basic moves in a dance, since the routines are each taught to a count of eight. Finally, don't concentrate on counting at the expense of your dancing. It is more important just to enjoy moving to the music.

A WORD ABOUT PREGNANCY

Bellydance is the original childbirth preparation both in its origins and in its movement principles. Many of the muscle isolation and relaxation techniques are similar to those taught in Lamaze classes. There are also psychological benefits to be gained from bellydancing during pregnancy—it can remind a woman that despite the radical changes her body is experiencing, she is still a sensual being. Having said this, you should consult your doctor before beginning and confirm that it is safe for you to bellydance.

MEDICAL CONSIDERATIONS

Bellydance is a safe and gentle exercise that can be practiced by people of any age and fitness level. However, as with any physical activity, listen to your body, and if you experience pain or discomfort, stop immediately.

BASIC STANCE

Now you are ready to begin bellydancing. For most of the basic moves, you begin in the Basic Stance. Start in this position, and try to maintain a poised, lifted, and elegant posture throughout your bellydance session.

• Stand with feet flat, hip-width apart, and your weight evenly distributed over both feet. Your knees should be slightly bent or "soft."

• Tilt your pelvis forward, tucking it under so that your back is straight, and squeeze in your buns (gluteal muscles). Use your lower abdominals to hold this position and prevent any unneccessary strain from being put on the lower back. This brings your focus to your center of gravity and to your core area: Your abdominals, buns, and hips.

• Lift your ribcage up and away from your hips by lengthening your abdominals. Feel the separation between your torso and hips that allows you freedom to move them independently of each other.

• Drop your shoulders down. Be sure to keep your neck and shoulders relaxed and your chin slightly lifted.

• Hold your hands as delicately as possible, relaxed but not limp, with fingers graceful and slightly separated. Sometimes when students concentrate on a more challenging move, I've noticed they actually make fists. Your hands complement the movements of your body; if they are tense and unexpressive, they will detract from the elegance of your movements.

Many of these points apply to your posture when you begin moving. Remember to try to remain proud and elegant when bellydancing.

The Basic Stance is your starting position for many of the basic moves. Stand relaxed but poised—key points for good posture in general.

lift chin slightly

keep neck relaxed

keep shoulders down and level

lengthen abdominals and lift ribcage

tuck pelvis under so that back is straight

relax hands and separate fingers slightly

bend knees slightly; don't lock legs straight

distribute weight evenly over both feet

feet are hip-width apart

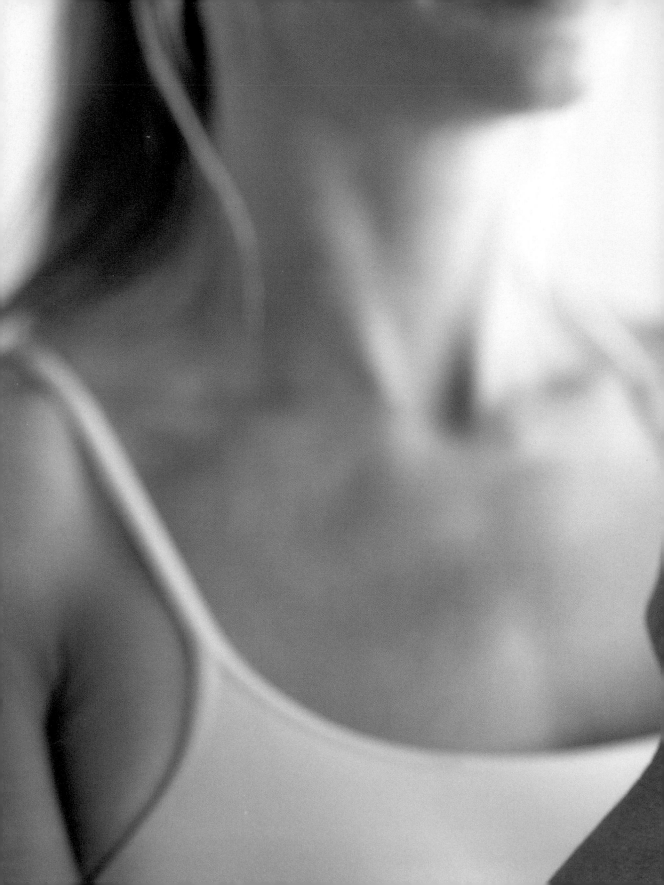

STRETCHING ROUTINE

Bellydance is a wonderful workout for the body but also for the mind and spirit. Take a few minutes to prepare for your practice by working through this tension-releasing sequence of stretches known as the Goddess Salutation. This routine introduces you to the movement principles unique to bellydance. They are the basis from which you will build the fluid, graceful, and controlled movements into a workout and even an art form.

GODDESS SALUTATION

This sequence of stretches is my way of preparing the body and the mind for a bellydance workout. I have included instructions on breathing where it is important to coordinate it with your movements, otherwise breathe deeply and regularly. Try to maintain a slow, steady pace as you move, flowing from one position to the next. At the end of the five minutes that it takes to complete the sequence, you'll find that you feel both relaxed and renewed and, most importantly, ready to begin bellydancing. Note that you can also perform the Goddess Salutation as a cool down at the end of your bellydance session.

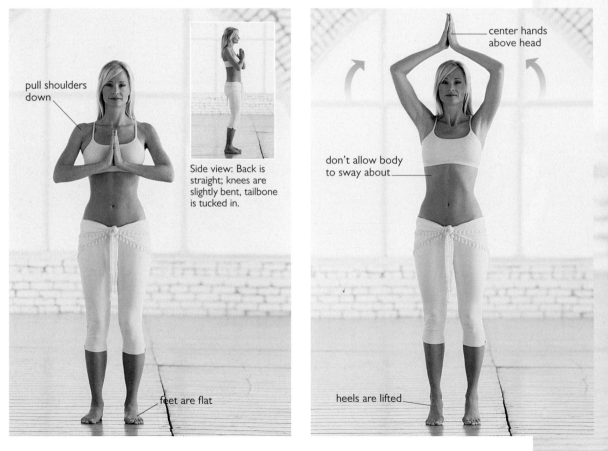

pull shoulders down

Side view: Back is straight; knees are slightly bent, tailbone is tucked in.

center hands above head

don't allow body to sway about

feet are flat

heels are lifted

1 Stand with feet hip-width apart, tailbone tucked in, and back straight. Hold your hands in praying position at your chest. Squeeze in your buns and lengthen your abdominals, lifting your ribcage.

2 Breathe in as you open your arms at your sides, then raise them so that your hands meet, palms together, above your head. As you do this, slowly lift your heels and find your center of balance.

relax neck
and shoulders

keep shoulders level

relax your hands

bend elbows slightly

bend both knees

3 Breathe out as you lower your hands, extending them at your sides. As you do this, bend your knees, being careful to keep your back straight and your hips tucked under.

4 Straighten your legs and bring your hands back up into praying position at your chest.

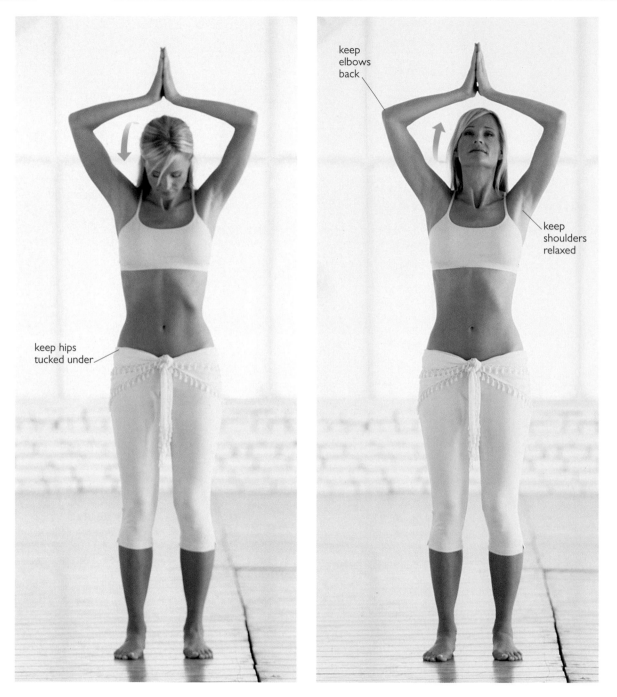

keep elbows back

keep shoulders relaxed

keep hips tucked under

5 Lift your hands up so that your palms meet above your head. Slowly lower your head forward. Feel the stretch along your spine as you take a deep breath in then slowly exhale.

6 Raise your head, then tilt it back, lifting your chin slightly. Take a deep breath in, then out. Be careful not to lean back—look diagonally up, not directly up.

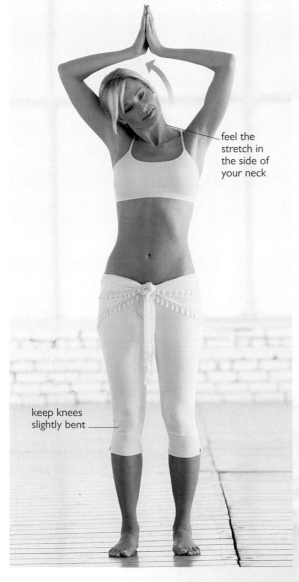

feel the
stretch in
the side of
your neck

use abdominals
to hold torso
in position

keep knees
slightly bent

7 Lower your head to the right side. Hold this
position for one breath in and one breath out.
Lower your head to the left, breathing in the same
way, then return to the center.

8 Slowly circle your head once to the right, taking
a deep breath in, then releasing it. Then circle
once to the left, breathing in the same way.

▶

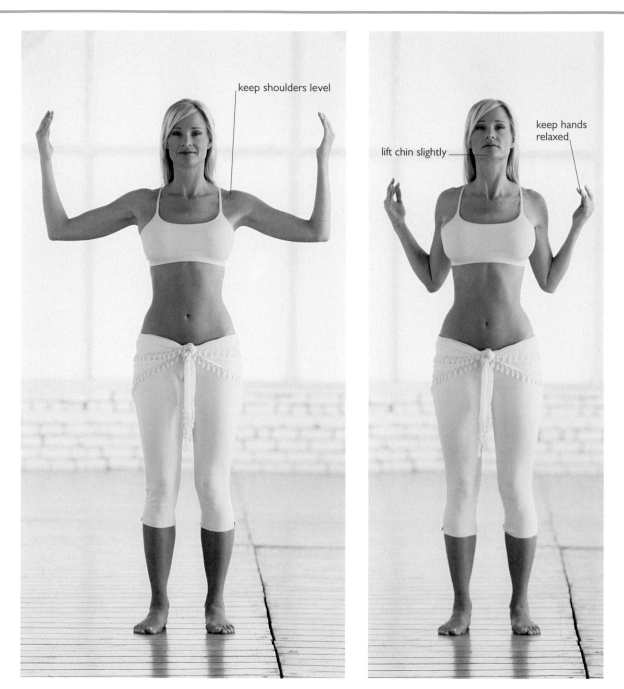

keep shoulders level

lift chin slightly

keep hands relaxed

9 With your head center, slowly lower your arms until your hands are at face level with palms facing in and your elbows are out at your sides. Feel the stretch in your upper arms. Be sure to keep your hips tucked under and your back straight.

10 Open your chest by pulling your shoulders back and squeezing your shoulder blades into your back as if trying to get your elbows to meet. Hold for one breath in and one breath out.

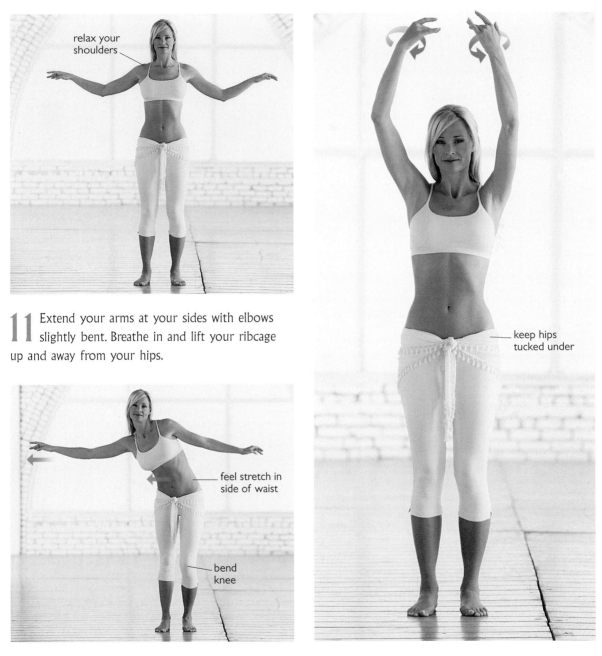

relax your
shoulders

keep hips
tucked under

feel stretch in
side of waist

bend
knee

11 Extend your arms at your sides with elbows slightly bent. Breathe in and lift your ribcage up and away from your hips.

12 Reach to the right with your right arm and slide your ribcage to the right. Feel the stretch in the left side of your waist. Increase the stretch by bending your left knee slightly. Hold for one breath cycle, then stretch the left side of your waist in the same way. Return to the center.

13 Raise your hands above your head, and rotate them inward 4 times at the wrists. Remember to relax your hands since they can often be tense, but keep your wrists strong. Be sure not to allow your arms to move around.

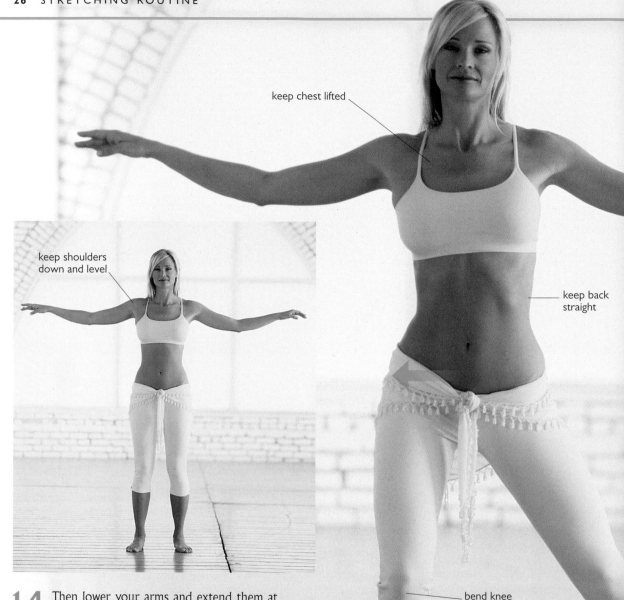

keep chest lifted

keep shoulders down and level

keep back straight

bend knee

toes on both feet point forward

14 Then lower your arms and extend them at your sides, being sure to keep them relaxed.

15 Step out to your right double hip-width with your right leg as you shift your weight onto your right leg, bend your right knee, and push your right hip out. Feel the stretch in your inner thigh. Breathe in, then out. Then shift your weight to the left side and repeat the stretch, pushing your left hip out. Finally, step your right foot in so that your feet are hip-width apart.

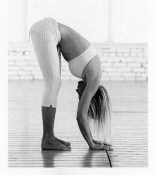

Side view: Knees are slightly bent; torso, shoulders, and arms are relaxed.

16 Bend forward from your hips. Relax your shoulders, and let your head and arms hang like a ragdoll. Be careful to keep your knees soft to prevent straining your lower back. Allow your weight to shift slightly forward onto your toes. As you breathe in then out, feel the stretch in the backs of your thighs (hamstrings).

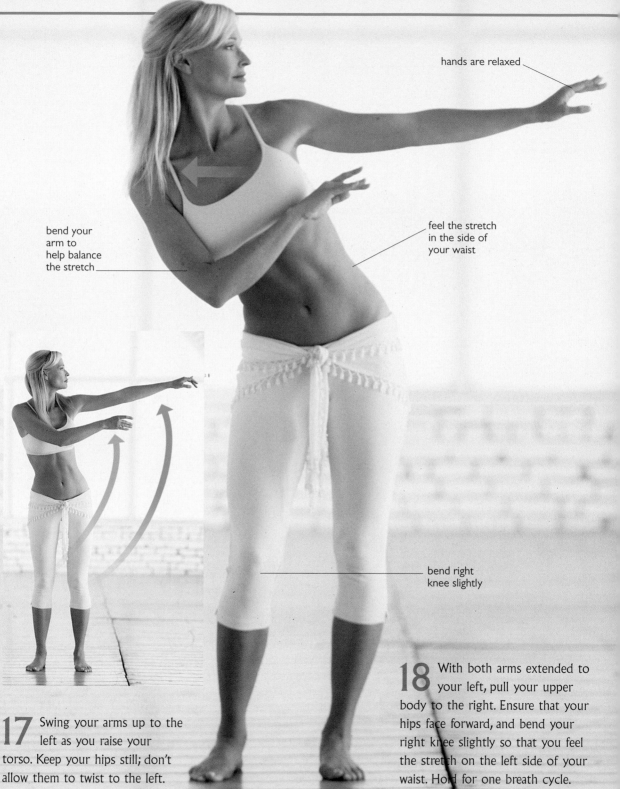

hands are relaxed

bend your
arm to
help balance
the stretch

feel the stretch
in the side of
your waist

bend right
knee slightly

17 Swing your arms up to the
left as you raise your
torso. Keep your hips still; don't
allow them to twist to the left.

18 With both arms extended to
your left, pull your upper
body to the right. Ensure that your
hips face forward, and bend your
right knee slightly so that you feel
the stretch on the left side of your
waist. Hold for one breath cycle.

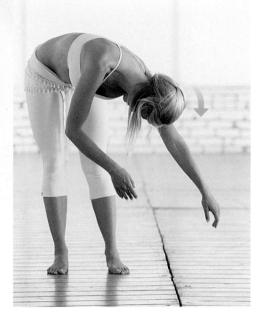

19 Reach to the left, swinging your arms down as you drop your torso back down to the center. Repeat steps 17 and 18 on the right side.

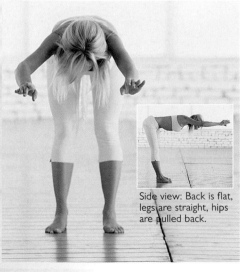

Side view: Back is flat, legs are straight, hips are pulled back.

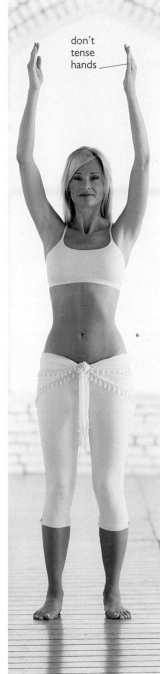

don't tense hands

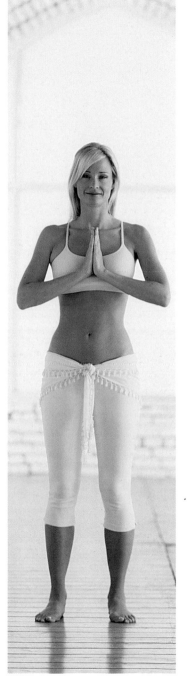

20 Use your lower abdominals to lift your torso and reach out in front of you. Try to keep your back flat.

21 Then reach up. Take a deep breath in, then slowly exhale.

22 Finish by bringing your hands together in the praying position at your chest.

QUICK REFERENCE

Once you are familiar with the stretches that make up the Goddess Salutation, refer to this quick-reference summary chart to help you perform the entire sequence. Remember, this routine can be performed as a warm up and also at the end of your session as a cool down.

Goddess Salutation

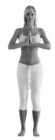

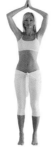

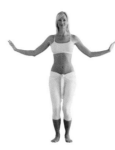

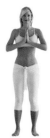

| 1. praying position
p20 | 2. raise arms
p20 | 3. lower arms
p21 | 4. praying position
p21 |

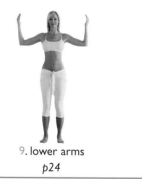

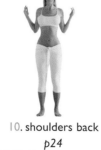

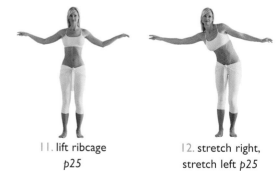

| 9. lower arms
p24 | 10. shoulders back
p24 | 11. lift ribcage
p25 | 12. stretch right,
stretch left *p25* |

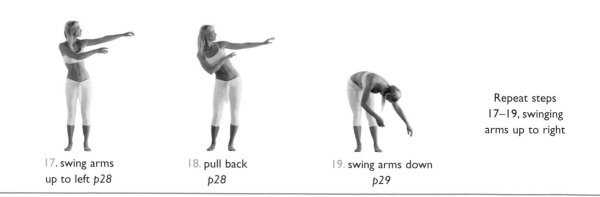

| 17. swing arms
up to left *p28* | 18. pull back
p28 | 19. swing arms down
p29 | Repeat steps
17–19, swinging
arms up to right |

*Freedom comes from a true
connection to your body.*

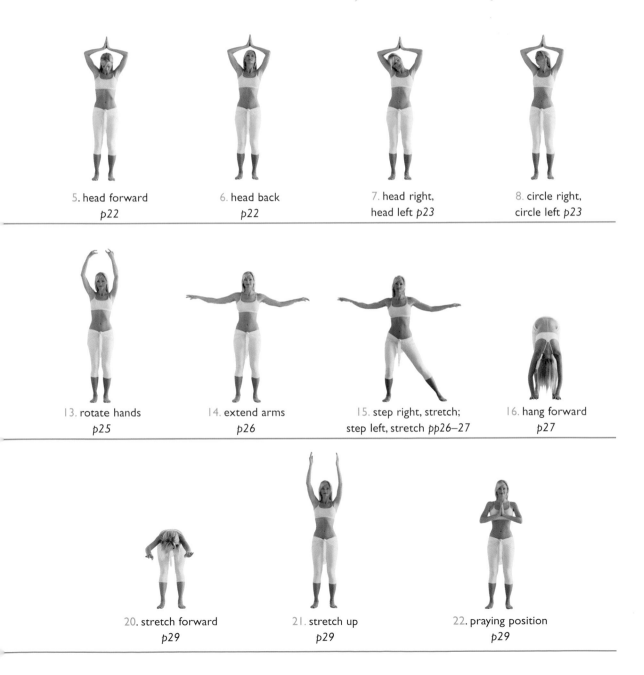

5. head forward
p22

6. head back
p22

7. head right,
head left *p23*

8. circle right,
circle left *p23*

13. rotate hands
p25

14. extend arms
p26

15. step right, stretch;
step left, stretch *pp26–27*

16. hang forward
p27

20. stretch forward
p29

21. stretch up
p29

22. praying position
p29

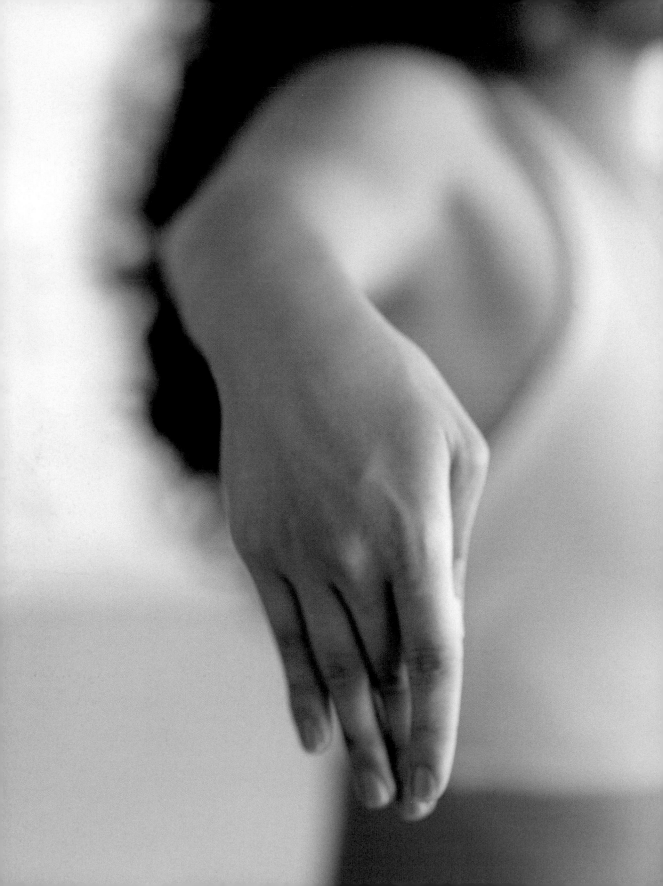

BASIC MOVES

LEVEL ONE

Enjoy the freedom that comes from making circles with your hips and swaying them from side to side. Discover the sensuous, willowy movements of Snake Arms. These classic bellydance moves may look simple, but you might be surprised by what a great workout they provide. Practice the moves on the pages that follow and have fun with them: Introduce feeling by moving slowly and smoothly, then quickly and sharply. Here you begin laying the foundations of your bellydance practice.

CLASSIC ARMS

As you begin learning the basic bellydance hip movements, you may feel more comfortable if you have something to do with your arms. This simple arm position announces your presence and adds grace to your movements. The raised arm catches the audience's attention, while the lower arm usually frames the moving hip. For example, in this position, you could perform a *Hip Lift and Drop* (see pp44–45) with your right hip.

keep neck and shoulders relaxed

lift chest

R aise one arm above your head, with palm facing out and fingers slightly parted and graceful. Hold the other arm down at your hip.

relax hands, but keep fingers graceful

TIPS AND TECHNIQUE

• Assume this pose with attitude. Stand proud; hold your head high.
• Add movement to this pose by rotating your hands inward as you fan your fingers.
• Combine this pose with *Hip Lifts and Drops*, *Tunisian Twists*, and *Moroccan Hip Circles*.

GENIE ARMS

This essential bellydance arm position draws attention to the chest and shoulder area as well as to the face. Think of yourself as a mischievous genie. Don't be tempted to hide behind your arms, hold your head high above them. When holding this arm position, be sure to keep your back straight and watch that you don't lean forward.

keep shoulders down and level

separate fingers slightly

keep hips tucked under

Cross your arms at chest level in front of your body so that your forearms are parallel. Be careful not to tense your neck and shoulders.

TIPS AND TECHNIQUE
• Maintain an even distance between your forearms when holding this pose.
• Combine Genie Arms with *Chest Lifts and Drops* and *Chest Slides* (see *Genie Dance, Part Two*).
• Try holding this arm position while performing slow *Chest Circles*.

SNAKE ARMS

This graceful, fluid movement appears to ripple across the body from one arm to the other. To begin with, practice with one arm at a time, then add the other arm and practice alternating them so that as you raise one arm, you lower the other. Make the movements large and undulating for dramatic effect, or simply ripple your arms at shoulder level (see *Small Snake Arms*, opposite). Snake Arms not only sculpts your upper body, it improves arm and shoulder flexibility.

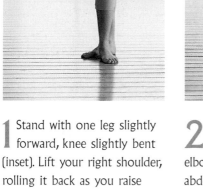

keep shoulder back

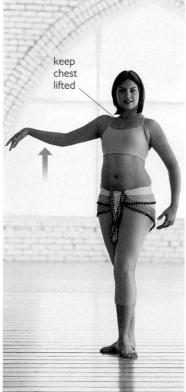

keep chest lifted

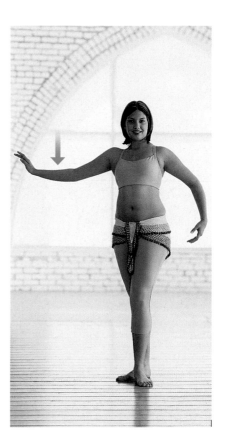

1 Stand with one leg slightly forward, knee slightly bent (inset). Lift your right shoulder, rolling it back as you raise your right elbow.

2 Lift your wrist up as you drop your shoulder and elbow slightly. Use your upper abdominals to keep your ribcage lifted and your torso straight.

3 Flick your wrist up, and lower your arm in the same order that you raised it: Shoulder, elbow, then wrist. Simultaneously begin raising your left arm in the same order.

"trail" your fingers
to add grace to
the movement

keep hips still
and tucked under

5 Practice raising and
lowering your arms in
opposition to create a fluid,
rhythmic movement. Be careful
not to allow your shoulders
to roll forward.

Workout Repetitions	
Beginner	4 times on each side
Intermediate	12 times on each side

SMALL SNAKE ARMS

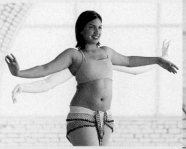

4 As you lower your right arm,
continue raising your left arm:
Shoulder first, then elbow and wrist.
Keep your back straight and your
hips tucked under.

Try this subtle variation of Snake
Arms, making the undulations
smaller. Ripple your arms at
shoulder level at your sides, keeping
the movements fluid and rhythmic.

CHEST SLIDE

This move clearly demonstrates one of the most important principles of bellydance: Muscle isolation. Imagine that your hips and torso are separate pieces, able to move independently of each other. Lengthen your abdominals and use them to move your chest while keeping your hips absolutely still. Mastering this move is essential for learning the *Chest Circle* (see pp74–75).

TIPS AND TECHNIQUE
• Wear a coin-fringed hip scarf, taking note that if you make a sound, you are moving your hips.
• Breathe in as you lengthen your abdominals and lift your chest.
• Feel this move in your upper and side abdominals.

Workout Repetitions	
Beginner	16 times in each direction
Intermediate	32 times in each direction

2 Then lengthen your abdominals in the same way to slide your chest across to the right. Keep the movement smooth, not sharp.

keep hips still

1 Begin in the *Basic Stance* (inset) with hands on hips. Keeping your hips still, breathe in, lengthen your abdominals, and slide your chest to the left.

CHEST LIFT AND DROP

The Chest Lift and Drop is very like a crunch, only better since it puts no stress at all on the neck or back. This move helps to build strength in the upper abdominals while also improving posture. When included in a dance routine, the accent can be on the lift or the drop. You might perform a dramatic Chest Drop to end a routine but never successive lifts and drops.

TIPS AND TECHNIQUE

• Breathe in as you lift your chest, breathe out as you drop it.
• Practice this move to help perfect technique for *Chest Circles* and *Chest Camels*.
• Feel this move in your upper and side abdominals.

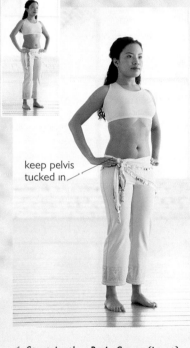

keep pelvis tucked in

2 Keeping your back straight, breathe out as you contract your upper abdominals and drop your ribcage.

don't allow shoulders to roll too far forward

1 Start in the *Basic Stance* (inset) with hands on hips. Lift your ribcage by breathing in and lengthening your upper abdominals.

Workout Repetitions	
Beginner	12 lifts and 12 drops
Intermediate	24 lifts and 24 drops

HIP SWAY

As its name suggests, the Hip Sway is a soft, smooth movement. It will familiarize you with the two basic techniques for moving your hips in bellydance: Bending your knees, and shifting your weight from one leg to the other. As you sway, allow your upper body and arms to follow the movement of your hips. Try to sway rhythmically and evenly from one side to the other; don't pause in the center or on one side. Think of palm trees swaying in a breeze.

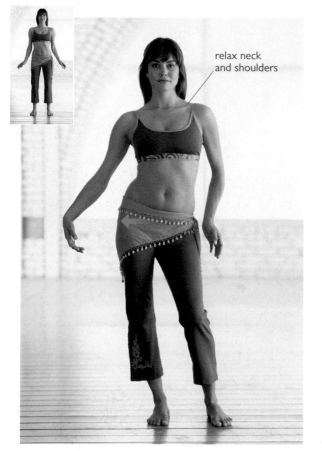

relax neck and shoulders

bend knee as you push out opposite hip

1 Begin in the *Basic Stance* (inset). Shift your weight onto your right leg as you push your right hip out to the side and bend your left knee slightly. Sway your arms to help you feel the movement in your hips.

2 Shift your weight onto your left leg as you push your left hip out to the side and bend your right knee slightly. Your knees move your hips; take care not to lift your heels as you sway.

keep shoulders
back and relaxed

keep
abdominals
contracted

Workout Repetitions	
Beginner	20 times in each direction
Intermediate	40 times in each direction

POINTS TO WATCH

• Be sure not to twist your upper body and shoulders as you move your hips.
• Keep your hips straight as you sway from side to side.
• Keep your knees soft, bending them slightly to move your hips.

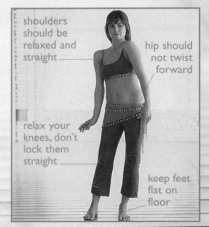

shoulders should be relaxed and straight

hip should not twist forward

relax your knees, don't lock them straight

keep feet flat on floor

3 Practice shifting your weight from one leg to the other, keeping both feet flat on the floor.

HIP POP

Very similar to the *Hip Sway* (see pp40–41), the Hip Pop also involves shifting your weight while bending your knees, but the movement is sharper and faster. You literally "pop" your hips from side to side, holding the position for one count rather than moving smoothly as for the Hip Sway. This provocative move is characteristic of the American Tribal bellydance style.

TIPS AND TECHNIQUE

• Wear a coin-fringed hip scarf or belt to help you hear the rhythm as you move your hips.
• Straighten your leg as you "pop" your hip to the side, but don't lock it straight.
• Feel this move in your inner and outer thighs and side abdominals.

leg is straight but not locked

be careful not to twist hip forward

1 Begin in the *Basic Stance* (inset). Shift your weight onto your right leg as you push your right hip out sharply to the side and bend your left knee.

2 Shift your weight onto your left leg as you push your left hip out sharply to the side and bend your right knee.

Workout Repetitions	
Beginner	12 times in each direction
Intermediate	36 times in each direction

HIP SHIMMY

This is one of the most challenging bellydance moves but also one of the most fun. It requires strength, flexibility, coordination, and endurance to generate the powerful vibrations of the Hip Shimmy. Part of the skill is building up speed and then maintaining it. Start with the *Hip Pop* (see opposite), and work up to a shimmy. Keep your knees loose and let your hips go—you'll be surprised by what an excellent cardiovascular workout you get from shimmying.

TIPS AND TECHNIQUE

• If you tighten up and "lose" your shimmy, slow down to the slower paced *Hip Pop*, then gradually work up speed again.
• Giggle as you jiggle; you'll feel other parts of your body moving too.
• Feel this move in the fronts of your thighs and your side abdominals.

Workout Repetitions	
Beginner	30 seconds
Intermediate	2 minutes

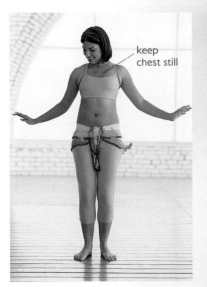

keep chest still

1 Start by practicing the *Hip Pop* (see opposite), then gradually speed up. Push your right hip to the right, bending your left knee, then push your left hip to the left, bending your right knee.

2 As you speed up, bend your knees less as you move your hips from side to side. Your knees generate the movement—almost like pistons—but it is your hips that vibrate. Remember to keep your chest still.

HIP LIFT AND DROP

When performing this sharp, dramatic hip movement, the accent can be on the lift, the drop, or both. A bellydancer will generally include one lift or drop in her routine for dramatic effect, or she might perform several in quick succession. The key is to focus the movement in the hips and not to allow your chest to move or your head to bob up and down. Hip Lifts and Drops are typical of the Modern Egyptian style of bellydance.

TIPS AND TECHNIQUE

• Firm your buns when practicing this move by contracting them as you lift your hip and relaxing them as you drop it.
• Feel this move in your buns, thighs, side abdominals (obliques), and the outer sides of your hips.

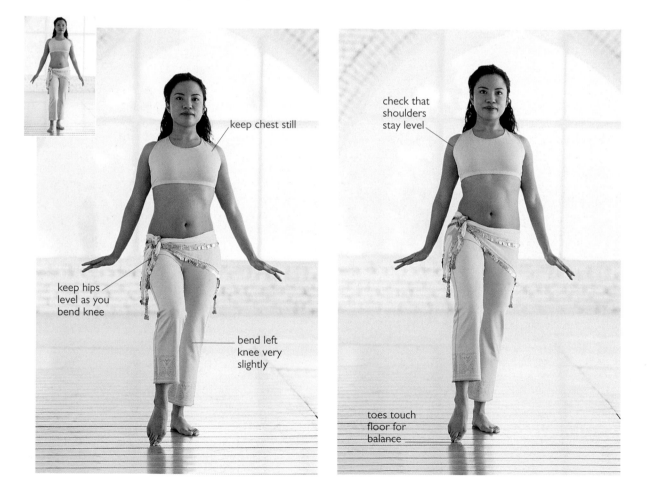

keep chest still

keep hips level as you bend knee

bend left knee very slightly

check that shoulders stay level

toes touch floor for balance

1 Stand with your right foot half a step further forward than your left, your weight on your left leg (inset). Lift your right heel and bend your right knee.

2 Raise your right hip by straightening your right leg and contracting your side abdominals. Be careful not to allow your chest and head to move.

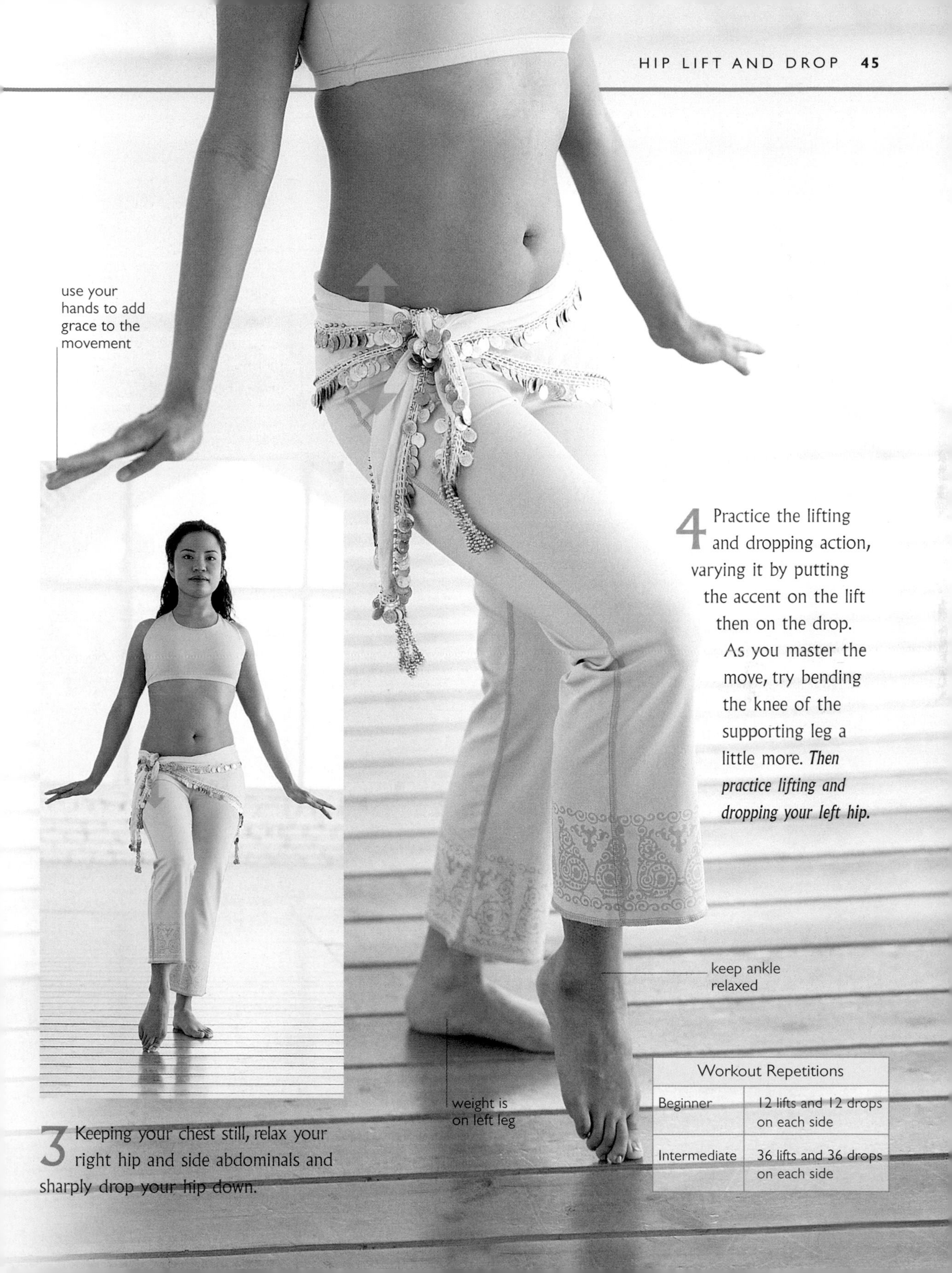

use your
hands to add
grace to the
movement

4 Practice the lifting
and dropping action,
varying it by putting
the accent on the lift
then on the drop.
As you master the
move, try bending
the knee of the
supporting leg a
little more. *Then
practice lifting and
dropping your left hip.*

keep ankle
relaxed

weight is
on left leg

3 Keeping your chest still, relax your
right hip and side abdominals and
sharply drop your hip down.

Workout Repetitions	
Beginner	12 lifts and 12 drops on each side
Intermediate	36 lifts and 36 drops on each side

SMALL HIP CIRCLE

This move is so fundamental to bellydance that you'll see it in every style, from Turkish and Modern Egyptian to Cabaret. The smooth, controlled movements will define your waist, increase flexibility in the hips, and diffuse tension in your lower back. Practice it correctly by generating the movement from your core abdominal muscles, but keep your knees bent to prevent putting pressure on the lower back. Keep the movement slow, fluid, and seamless.

TIPS AND TECHNIQUE

- Try putting your hands on your hips to help you feel the muscles working.
- Isolate your chest, focusing on keeping it still, to lengthen and tone your abdominals.
- Feel this move in your lower abdominals and in your hips, buns, and thigh muscles.

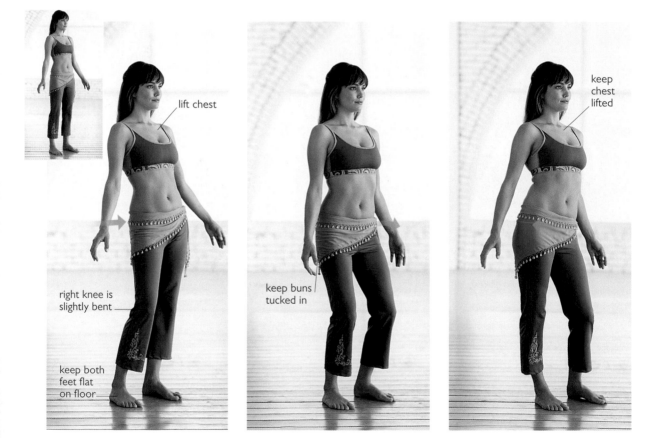

lift chest

right knee is slightly bent

keep both feet flat on floor

keep buns tucked in

keep chest lifted

1 Begin in the *Basic Stance* (inset). Shift your weight onto your left leg as you bend your right knee and smoothly push your left hip out to the left.

2 Shift your weight forward onto your toes, and bend both knees slightly. Keep your hips straight as you push your abdominals out.

3 Shift your weight onto your right leg, and bend your left knee as you push your right hip out to the right. Keep the movements smooth.

Workout Repetitions	
Beginner	8 times in each direction
Intermediate	24 times in each direction

relax your
shoulders

keep chest as
still as possible

weight is
evenly
distributed
over both feet

keep knees soft

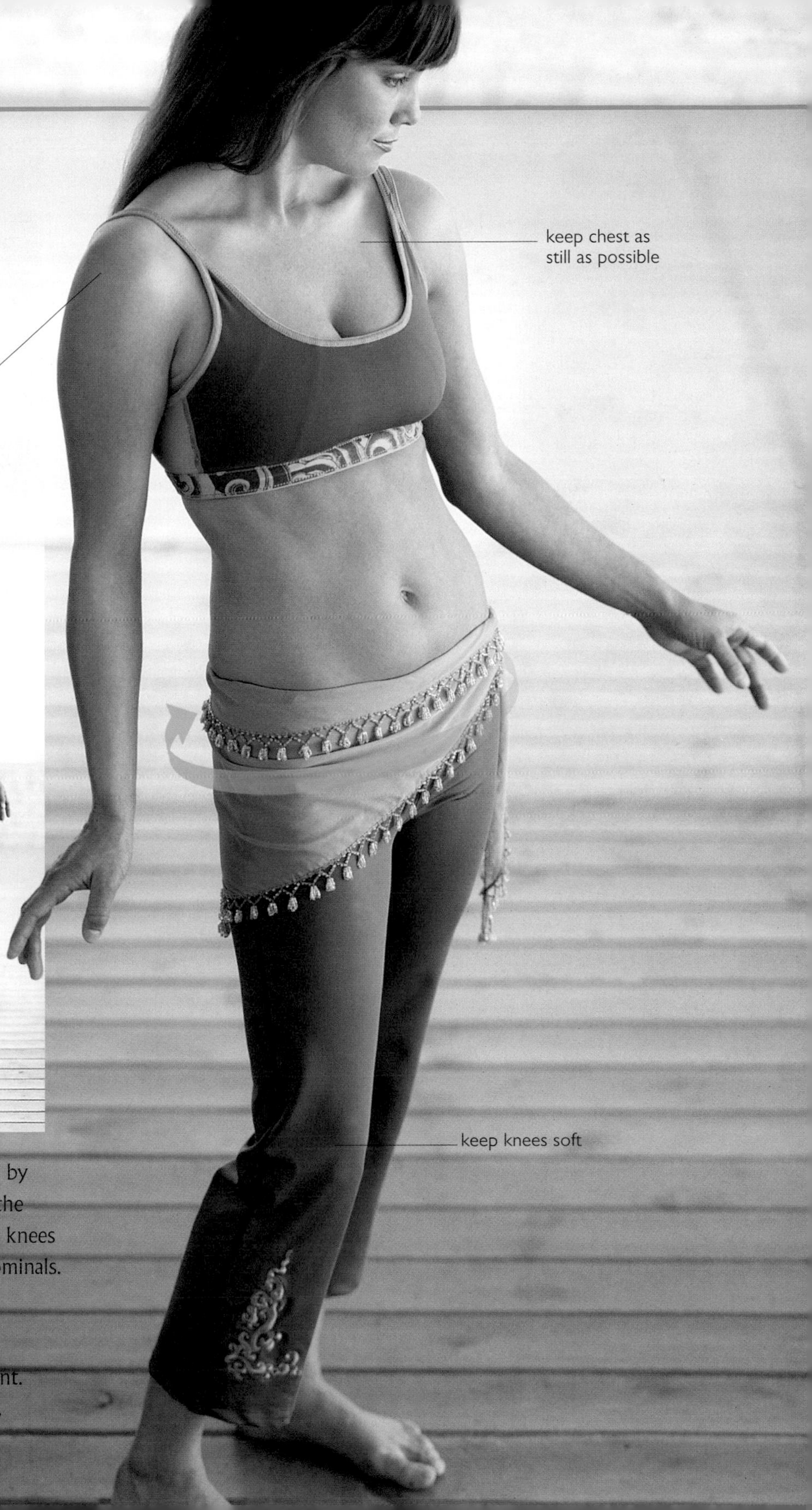

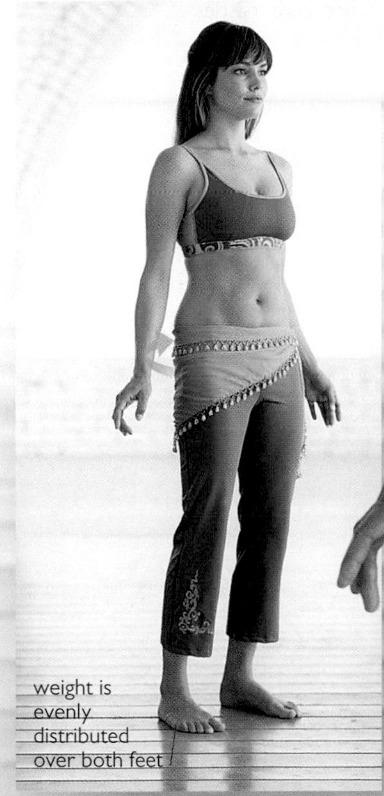

4 Complete the Hip Circle by
shifting your weight to the
center as you straighten your knees
and contract your lower abdominals.

5 Combine steps 1–4 in a
smooth, circular movement.
Practice circling in both directions.

LARGE HIP CIRCLE

This is without a doubt the best move for increasing flexibility in the hips. Pregnant students tell me that it feels wonderful to practice it, since it also helps to relax the lower back. Control the movement with your quads, the muscles at the fronts of your thighs. Move slowly and smoothly, and try raising your arms slightly at your sides to help you control the circular movement. When dancing, perform a single Large Hip Circle for dramatic effect.

TIPS AND TECHNIQUE

• Practice this move as a short warm-up exercise on its own: Hold each step for 5 seconds, feeling the stretch in your thighs. Then circle in the other direction, stretching in the same way.
• Feel this move working your inner and outer thigh muscles as well as your hips and buns.

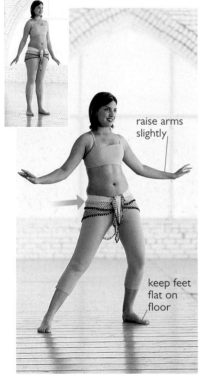

raise arms slightly

keep feet flat on floor

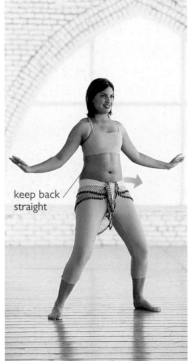

keep back straight

1 Begin in the *Basic Stance* (inset), then step out to the side with your left foot so that your feet are double hip-width apart. Bend your left knee as you push your left hip out to the left.

2 Bend both knees as you shift your weight forward and push your hips forward. Use your lower abdominals and quads to keep your back straight. Keep your chest lifted and your shoulders relaxed.

3 Shift your weight onto your right leg, and bend your right knee as you push your right hip out to the right. You should feel the stretch along the inside of your left thigh.

Workout Repetitions	
Beginner	4 times in each direction
Intermediate	10 times in each direction

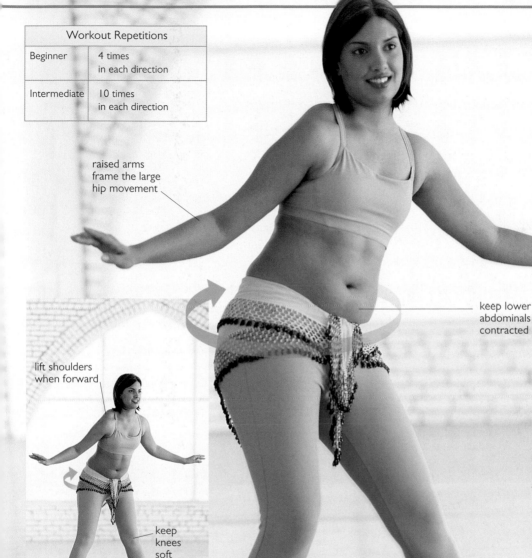

raised arms frame the large hip movement

keep lower abdominals contracted

lift shoulders when forward

keep knees soft

4 Complete the Large Hip Circle by straightening your right knee as you push your hips back. Be careful to keep your back flat and your shoulders and head lifted as you lean forward.

5 Combine steps 1–4 in a smooth, circular movement, being careful to keep your feet flat on the floor. *Then practice this move circling slowly in the opposite direction.*

MOROCCAN HIP CIRCLE

This sensual movement combines skills learned in the *Small Hip Circle* (see pp46–47), *Large Hip Circle* (see pp48–49), and the *Hip Lift and Drop* (see pp44–45). The aim is to keep the upper body still as you twist your hip forward, lift it, then circle it back and drop it. You can circle forward or back, but focus the movement in your hips, and don't allow your head to bob up and down. This move is more effective at tightening and lifting your buns than squats.

TIPS AND TECHNIQUE

• Try to form a perfect circle with your hip—people tend to twist further forward than back.
• Keep your chest still in order to tone and sculpt the side abdominals more effectively.
• Feel this move in your buns, side abdominals, and thighs.

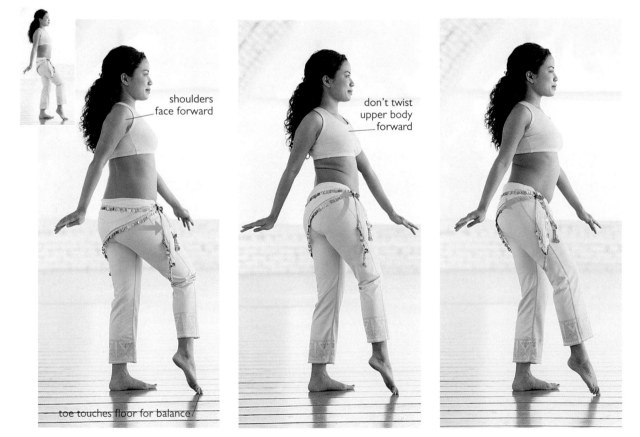

shoulders face forward

don't twist upper body forward

toe touches floor for balance

1 Begin with your weight on your left leg, your right foot slightly further forward than your left with heel lifted and knee slightly bent (inset). Twist your right hip forward.

2 With your hip still twisted forward, lift it by contracting your side abdominals and straightening your leg. Keep the movement smooth and controlled.

3 With your hip still lifted, slowly twist it round and back. Be careful not to allow your shoulders and upper body to twist back.

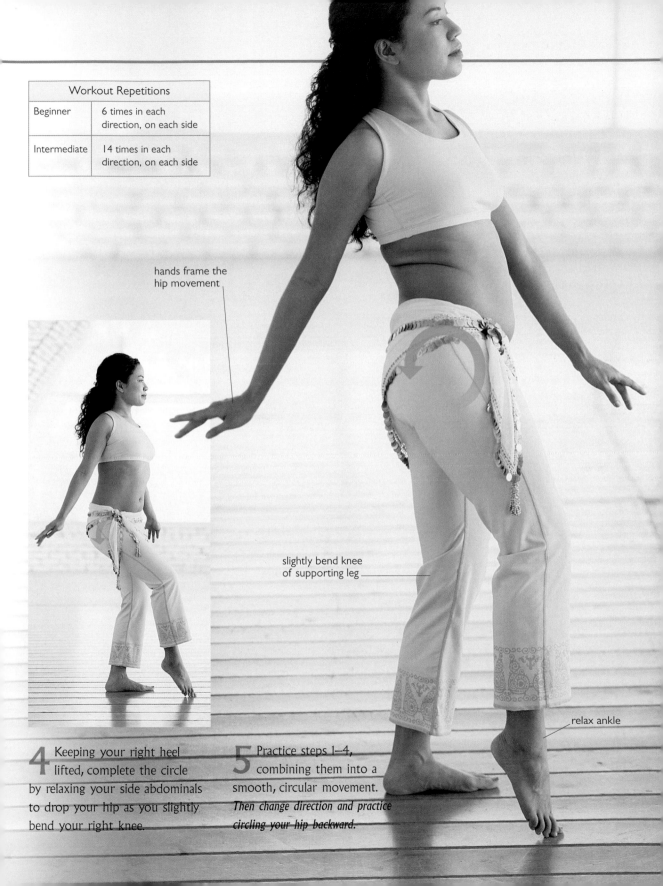

Workout Repetitions	
Beginner	6 times in each direction, on each side
Intermediate	14 times in each direction, on each side

hands frame the
hip movement

slightly bend knee
of supporting leg

relax ankle

4 Keeping your right heel lifted, complete the circle by relaxing your side abdominals to drop your hip as you slightly bend your right knee.

5 Practice steps 1–4, combining them into a smooth, circular movement. *Then change direction and practice circling your hip backward.*

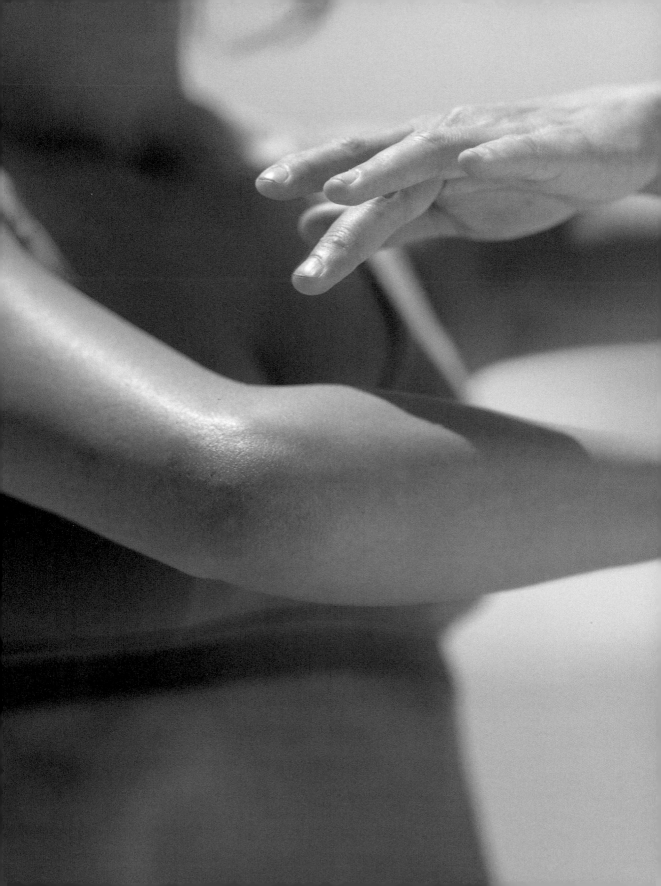

DANCE ROUTINE

LEVEL ONE

In the pages that follow I introduce a simple dance routine that links together movements learned in Basic Moves Level One. Here is your opportunity to practice shifting your weight and making transitions from one move to another, all while keeping a rhythm. The dance is presented in three parts, each consisting of an eight-count sequence. Choose some music with a regular rhythm and perform each step in time with the beat.

Tie on a hip scarf and let yourself go!

GENIE DANCE, PART ONE

Here you combine hip and arm movements for the first time in a dance. Keep the rhythm as you coordinate lifting your hip with rotating your hands at the start of the routine. Turn a little to your left to perform this sequence, so you face your audience at a slight angle and draw attention to the dramatic hip movements.

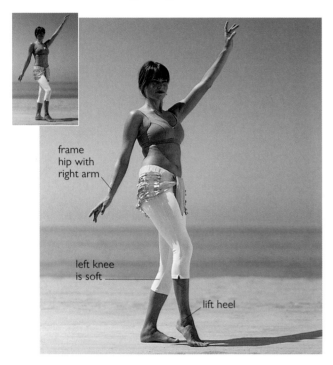

frame
hip with
right arm

left knee
is soft

lift heel

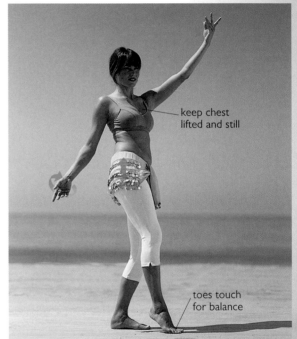

keep chest
lifted and still

toes touch
for balance

1 Begin with your right foot forward, your weight on your left leg, and your right knee slightly bent. Position your arms in *Classic Arms* with your right arm at your side (inset). On the beat, perform a dramatic *Hip Lift* with your right hip, then release it.

2 Repeat the *Hip Lift* with your right hip, accenting the lift on the beat by making it strong and sharp. As you lift your hip, rotate your hands inward and fan your fingers. Then release your hip.

At a glance

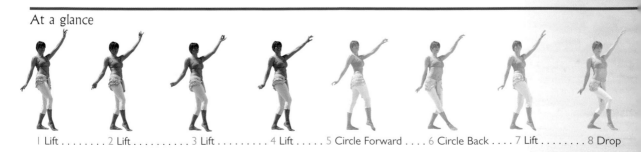

I Lift . . . . 2 Lift . . . . 3 Lift . . . . 4 Lift . . . . . 5 Circle Forward . . . . 6 Circle Back . . . . 7 Lift . . . . 8 Drop

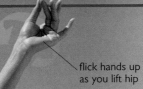

flick hands up
as you lift hip

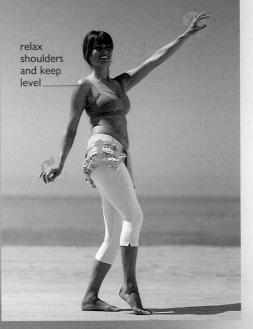

relax
shoulders
and keep
level

continue to rotate
hands inward

3 Perform another
sharp *Hip Lift* with
your right hip. Continue
to rotate your hands,
flicking them up as you
lift your hip. Then
release your hip.

4 Perform a final, dramatic *Hip Lift* with
your right hip. Then release your hip,
keeping your right heel slightly lifted in
preparation for the *Moroccan Hip Circle*.

keep heel lifted

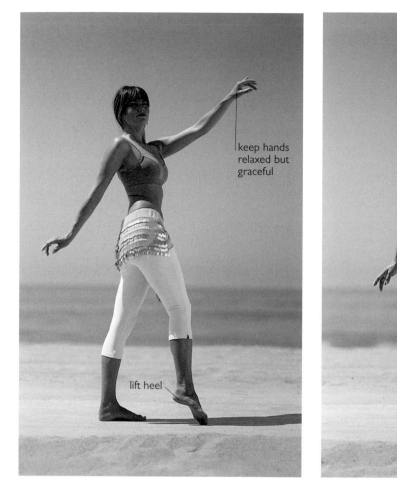

keep hands
relaxed but
graceful

lift heel

heel does
not touch
ground

5 Maintain the *Classic Arms* position, but stop rotating your hands, and focus attention on your hip. With your weight still on your left leg, begin a *Moroccan Hip Circle* by twisting your right hip forward then lifting it. Don't allow your upper body to twist forward as you circle your hip.

6 Complete the *Moroccan Hip Circle* by twisting your right hip back, then smoothly releasing it. Control the movement with your side abdominals. Keep your shoulders level.

At a glance

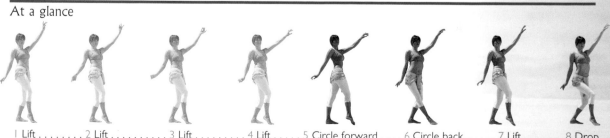

1 Lift . . . . 2 Lift . . . . 3 Lift . . . . 4 Lift . . . . . 5 Circle forward . . . . 6 Circle back. . . . . . 7 Lift . . . . 8 Drop

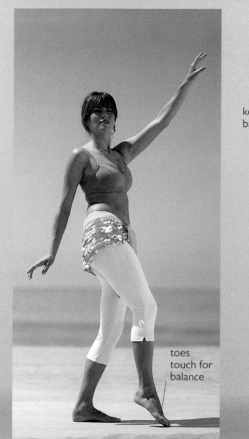

keep shoulders
back and relaxed

keep hands
relaxed and
graceful

toes
touch for
balance

7 Keeping your arms in the same position, shift your weight onto your left leg and perform a sharp *Hip Lift* on the right side.

bend knee of
supporting
leg slightly

8 Finish the routine by performing a sharp *Hip Drop* as you dramatically release your right hip.

weight is
on left leg

GENIE DANCE, PART TWO

In this eight-count sequence you make your first transition from an arm movement, *Snake Arms*, to a hip movement, the *Small Hip Circle*. The key is to keep your hips still as you move your chest. Have fun with this playful sequence, and once you have learned it, add it to Part One and practice the two together.

keep chest lifted

keep hips tucked under

weight is evenly distributed over both feet

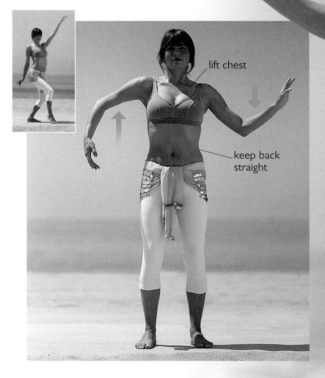

lift chest

keep back straight

1 From the *Hip Drop* with arms in *Classic Arms* pose (inset), lower your right heel and step forward with your left foot so you face your audience. With feet hip-width apart, raise your right arm as you begin lowering your left, and perform a *Small Snake Arm* at shoulder height, keeping the movement fluid.

2 Then perform a *Small Snake Arm* with your left arm, gracefully lowering your right arm as you raise your left one. Keep your chest lifted.

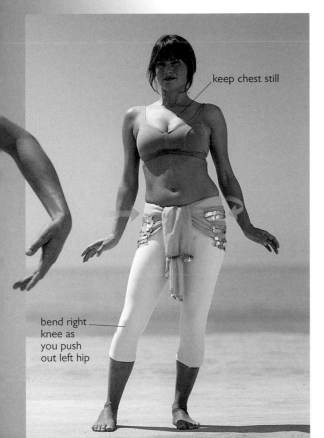

keep chest still

bend right knee as you push out left hip

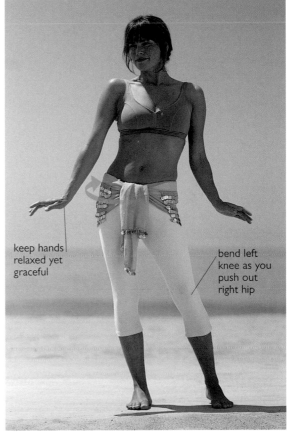

keep hands relaxed yet graceful

bend left knee as you push out right hip

3 Gracefully lower your arms to your sides as you shift your weight onto your left leg and begin a *Small Hip Circle* by bending your right knee and pushing your left hip out to the side in a smooth movement. Begin shifting your weight to the center, bending both knees.

4 Complete the *Small Hip Circle* by shifting your weight onto your right leg, bending your left knee, and smoothly pushing your right hip out to the side. Focus the movement on your hips by keeping your chest still as you then shift your weight to the center and straighten your legs.

At a glance

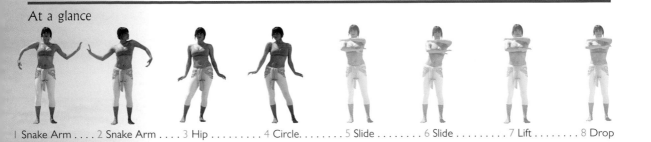

1 Snake Arm . . . . 2 Snake Arm . . . . 3 Hip . . . . 4 Circle. . . . . 5 Slide . . . . 6 Slide . . . . 7 Lift . . . . 8 Drop

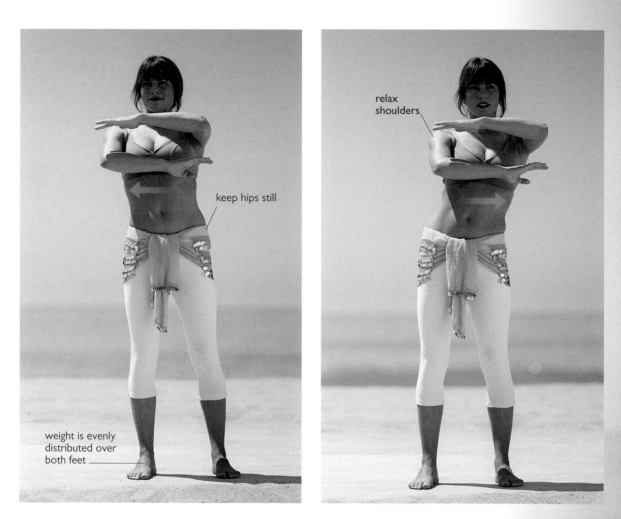

relax
shoulders

keep hips still

weight is evenly
distributed over
both feet

5 Move your arms into *Genie Arms,* positioning
your left forearm just above your right
at chest height. On the beat, perform a *Chest Slide*
to the right Remember to keep your shoulders level.

6 Perform a *Chest Slide* to the left on the beat.
Then slide your chest back to the center.
Keep your hips as still as possible to make the
chest movement appear more dramatic.

At a glance

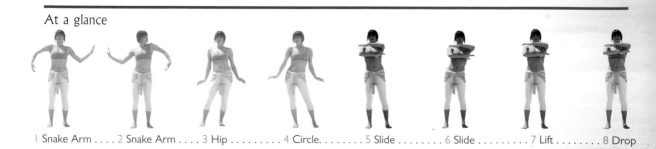

I Snake Arm . . . . 2 Snake Arm . . . . 3 Hip . . . . 4 Circle. . . . . 5 Slide . . . . 6 Slide . . . . 7 Lift . . . . 8 Drop

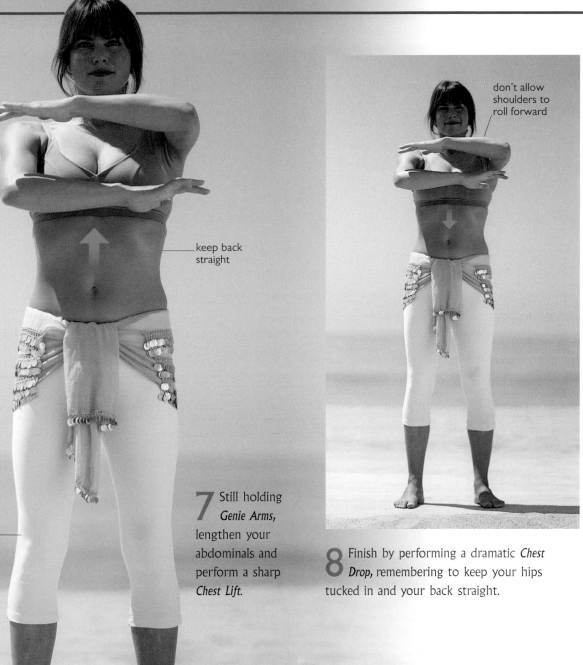

don't allow
shoulders to
roll forward

keep back
straight

ep
ees
t

7 Still holding
Genie Arms,
lengthen your
abdominals and
perform a sharp
Chest Lift.

8 Finish by performing a dramatic *Chest Drop,* remembering to keep your hips tucked in and your back straight.

GENIE DANCE FINALE

In this sequence I introduce some simple arm movements to be combined with hip movements that you learned in Basic Moves Level One. When you begin learning this sequence, concentrate on mastering the footwork, then when you feel confident, add the arms. Finally, add this sequence to the first two and practice the entire routine.

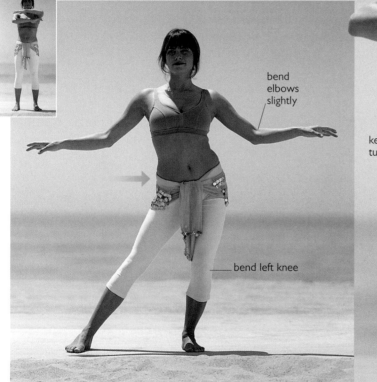

bend elbows slightly

bend left knee

keep hips tucked under

both knees are bent

feet are flat on ground

1 From the *Chest Drop* with *Genie Arms*, feet hip-width apart (inset), step out to the side with your right foot. Begin a *Large Hip Circle* to the right by shifting your weight onto your left leg and pushing your left hip out to the side. Extend your arms at your sides.

2 In a smooth movement, continue the *Large Hip Circle*, shifting your weight forward. Bring your hands together at chest level with fingertips facing each other, palms down, and elbows bent.

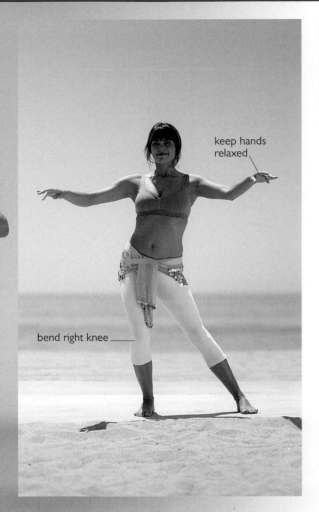

keep hands relaxed

bend right knee

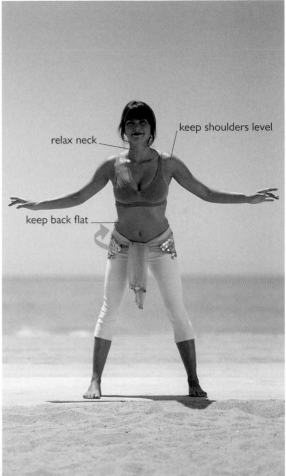

relax neck

keep shoulders level

keep back flat

3 Continue the *Large Hip Circle* by shifting your weight onto your right leg and pushing your right hip out to the side. Simultaneously begin extending your arms out at your sides.

4 Complete the *Large Hip Circle* by straightening your legs and pushing your hips back. As you do this, fully extend your arms at your sides. Keep your head lifted.

At a glance

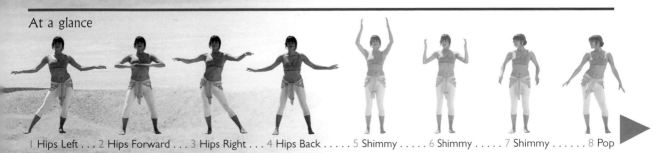

1 Hips Left . . . 2 Hips Forward . . . 3 Hips Right . . . 4 Hips Back . . . . . 5 Shimmy . . . . . 6 Shimmy . . . . . 7 Shimmy . . . . . . 8 Pop

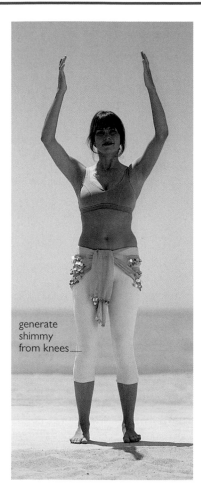

generate
shimmy
from knees

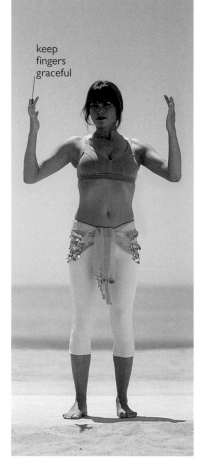

keep
fingers
graceful

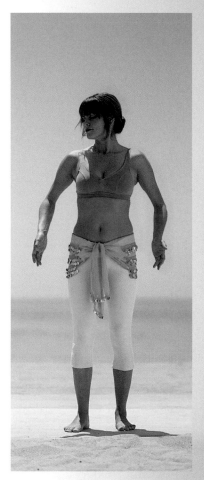

5 Step in with your right foot so feet are hip-width apart. Lift your hands above your head and *Hip Shimmy* by bending your knees slightly and rhythmically shaking your hips from side to side.

6 Slowly bring your hands down to shoulder level as you continue to perform a rhythmic *Hip Shimmy*.

7 Slowly bring your hands down to your hips, following the contours of your body as you *Hip Shimmy*.

At a glance

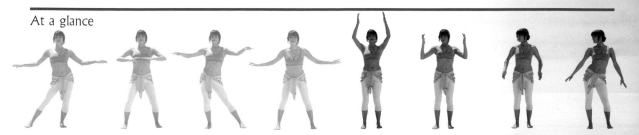

1 Hips Left . . . 2 Hips Forward . . . 3 Hips Right . . . 4 Hips Back . . . . . 5 Shimmy . . . . . 6 Shimmy . . . . . 7 Shimmy . . . . . . 8 Pop

keep shoulders level

flick out hands

bend knee slightly

8 Finish by performing a sharp *Hip Pop* with your right hip as you flick your hands out at your sides and assume your dramatic end pose.

GENIE DANCE SUMMARY

Once you've learned the three eight-count sequences that make up the first dance routine, refer to this chart to help you to link the routines together and perform the entire dance. Where helpful, I have indicated moves on the right with an "R" and moves on the left with an "L."

Genie Dance, Part One

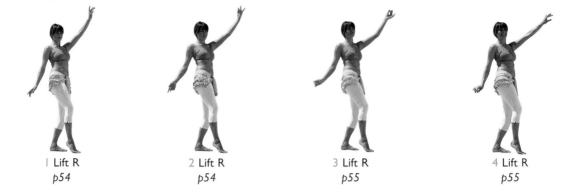

| 1 Lift R | 2 Lift R | 3 Lift R | 4 Lift R |
| p54 | p54 | p55 | p55 |

Genie Dance, Part Two

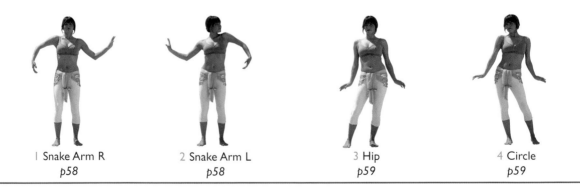

| 1 Snake Arm R | 2 Snake Arm L | 3 Hip | 4 Circle |
| p58 | p58 | p59 | p59 |

Genie Dance Finale

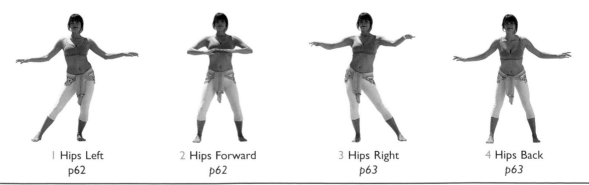

| 1 Hips Left | 2 Hips Forward | 3 Hips Right | 4 Hips Back |
| p62 | p62 | p63 | p63 |

Discover your own natural rhythm and grace.

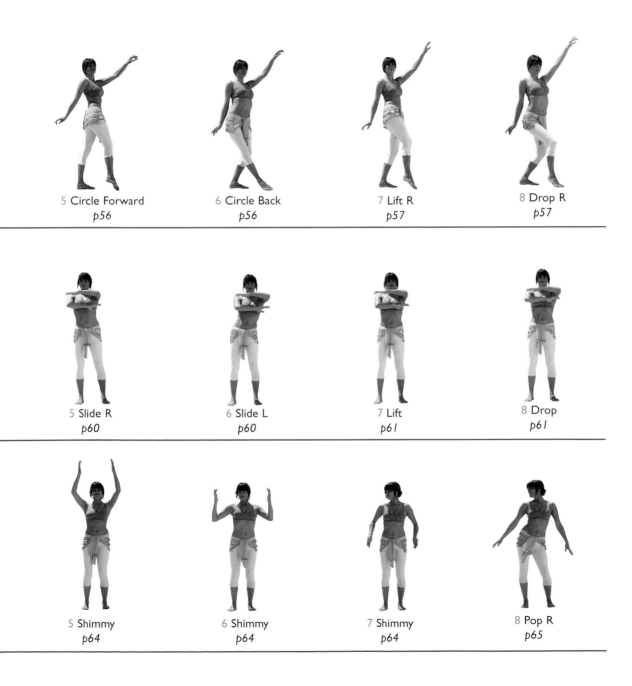

5 Circle Forward *p56*	6 Circle Back *p56*	7 Lift R *p57*	8 Drop R *p57*
5 Slide R *p60*	6 Slide L *p60*	7 Lift *p61*	8 Drop *p61*
5 Shimmy *p64*	6 Shimmy *p64*	7 Shimmy *p64*	8 Pop R *p65*

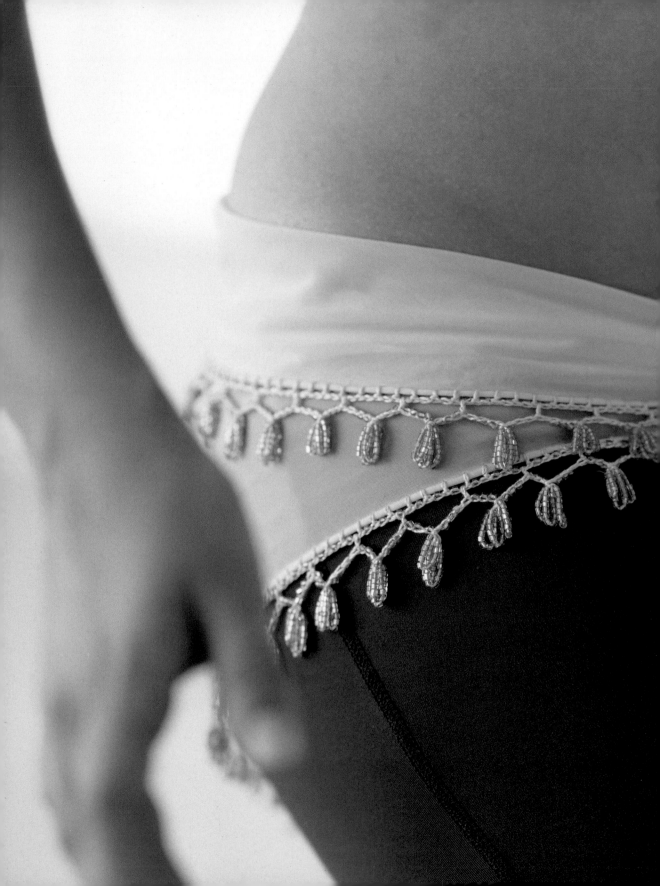

BASIC MOVES
LEVEL TWO

In Level Two, you build on skills learned in Basic Moves Level One. Here you learn fluid, sensuous hip movements that require more complex weight-shifting, such as the Figure Eight and the Hip Snake. Not only do you learn variations of basic moves such as Snake Arms, you learn how to combine them with traveling. Don't rush through these moves; focus on learning the breakdowns. It takes practice to perfect the muscle isolations and subtle coordination that make each movement appear effortless, graceful, and smooth.

GODDESS ARMS

Assume this simple arm position and you will immediately feel like a proud goddess. When combining Goddess Arms with a hip movement, place your hand on the moving hip to help draw attention to it. So, for example, in the position demonstrated here you could perform a *Hip Lift and Drop* (see pp44–45) with your left hip. Typical of the Cabaret bellydance style, this arm position adds instant glamour to the simplest of hip movements.

TIPS AND TECHNIQUE

• Hold your head high and look forward proudly.
• Combine Goddess Arms with the *Traveling Hip Lift and Drop*, and practice alternating your hand positions as you lift your hip (see *Goddess Dance, Part One*).

keep shoulders level

keep chest lifted

keep hand relaxed

Place one hand on your hip, the other just behind your head with elbow out to the side. Lift your chest, and keep your back straight.

ISIS ARMS

This is essentially *Small Snake Arms* (see p37) performed with one arm. The movement should be flowing and graceful and appear to be effortless—in fact, it isn't at all and provides a fantastic workout for the arms. For Isis Arms workout repetitions, follow the suggested workout repetitions for *Snake Arms* on page 37.

TIPS AND TECHNIQUE
• Combine Isis Arms with the *Hip Snake*; the undulating hip movements echo the fluid arm movements (see *Goddess Dance, Part Two*).
• Feel this move in your upper arms (triceps and biceps) as well as your upper back and shoulders.

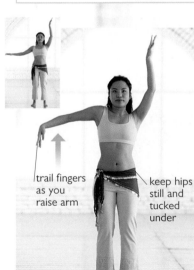

trail fingers as you raise arm

keep hips still and tucked under

keep elbow soft

1 Raise your left arm above your head with palm facing outward, and extend your right arm at shoulder height (inset). Lift your right shoulder, elbow, then wrist, as if performing a *Small Snake Arm.*

2 Flick your hand up, then slowly lower your shoulder, elbow, then wrist.

3 Repeat steps 1 and 2, undulating your arm at shoulder height at your side. Make the movements as smooth and graceful as possible. *Then practice Isis arms with your left arm.*

MERMAID ARMS

This movement is similar to *Snake Arms* (see pp36–37), except that here the flowing arm movements are performed in front of the body. These graceful arm undulations should be performed slowly for maximum effect—imagine that you are moving your arms underwater. For a dramatic effect, keep the arm movements large; for a more playful effect, make smaller, graceful hand movements at chest level (see *Small Mermaid Arms*, opposite).

TIPS AND TECHNIQUE

• Keep hands and fingers relaxed, but not limp, to add grace and expression to your movements.
• Try combining Mermaid Arms with *Hip Camels*.
• Feel this movement in your upper arms (biceps and triceps).

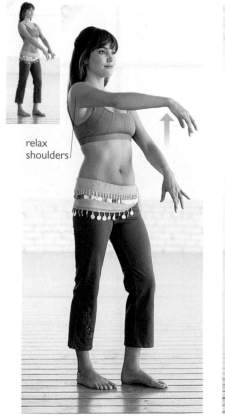

relax shoulders

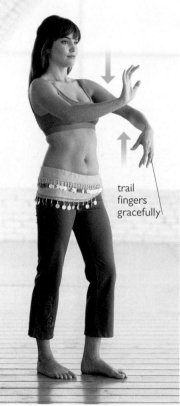

trail fingers gracefully

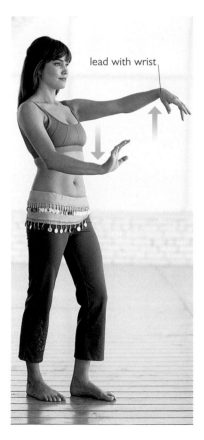

lead with wrist

1 Start with arms down and in front of your body with palms facing downward (inset). Raise your right arm to chest level in front of you, leading with your wrist.

2 Turn your right hand up and slowly lower your arm, bending your elbow slightly as you begin gracefully raising your left arm, leading with the wrist.

3 Continue slowly lowering your right arm as you raise your left arm to chest level in front of you. Keep your hands and fingers relaxed.

relax neck
and shoulders

keep hands relaxed
and graceful

keep hips still
and tucked under

Workout Repetitions	
Beginner	6 times on each arm
Intermediate	24 times on each arm

4 Repeat steps 1–3,
undulating your
arms in front of you.
As you raise one arm
to chest level, lower
the other to
approximately hip level.
Keep the movements
smooth and rhythmic.

SMALL MERMAID ARMS

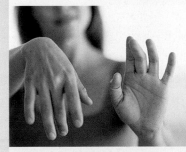

For a more subtle, playful effect,
make the movements smaller.
Undulate your arms at chest
level in front of you, and focus
more on your hands. As you raise
one hand, lower the other. The
movements can be slow or fast
but always graceful and rhythmic.

CHEST CIRCLE

Here you build on the abdominal skills learned in the *Chest Slide* (see p38) and the *Chest Lift and Drop* (see p39), combining the moves to make a smooth circle with your torso. Very few movements outside of bellydance require you to lengthen your abdominals in this way. You may find that your muscles are a bit tight to begin with, and it may take practice to achieve the smooth, fluid movement that makes this classic Cabaret-style move look so impressive.

TIPS AND TECHNIQUE

• Make this move more challenging by taking your hands off your hips as you practice it.
• Breathe in as you lift your chest, breathe out as you drop it.
• Feel this move in your upper abdominals, chest, and upper back.

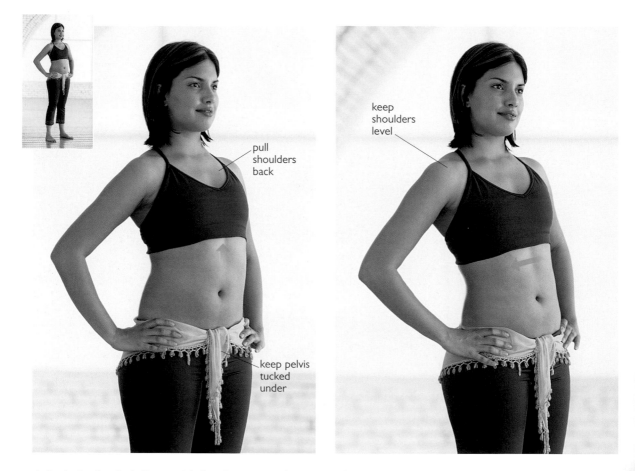

pull shoulders back

keep pelvis tucked under

keep shoulders level

1 Begin in the *Basic Stance* with hands on your hips to help you keep them still (inset). Lift your ribcage by lengthening your abdominals and stretching your torso up. Be careful not to push your chest out.

2 Maintaining the lifted position, slide your ribcage to the right. Ensure that you keep your hips still.

keep shoulders back

avoid locking knees straight

3 Drop your ribcage by contracting your upper abdominals. Be careful not to roll your shoulders forward.

4 With your ribcage still in the dropped position, and being careful to keep your hips still, slide your ribcage to the left.

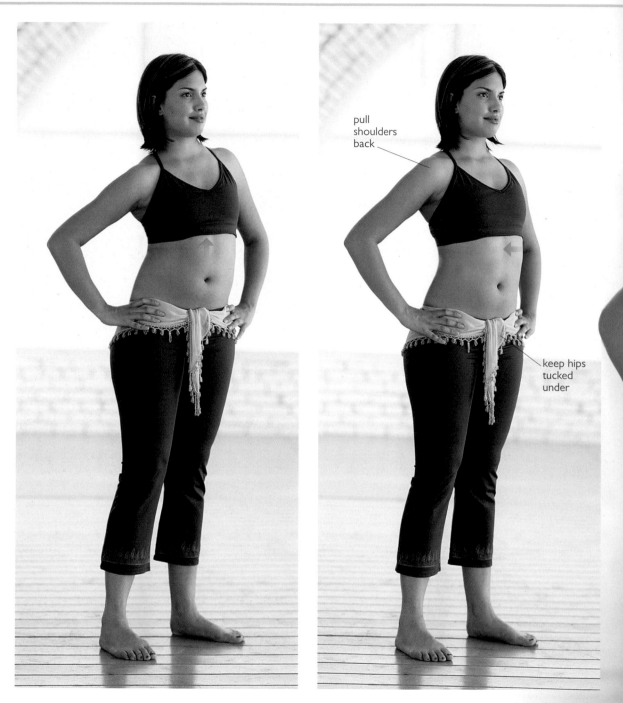

pull
shoulders
back

keep hips
tucked
under

5 With your ribcage still to the left, lift it by lengthening your abdominals. Remember to keep the movements smooth.

6 Still in the lifted position, slide your ribcage to the center. Keep your chest lifted and your shoulders back.

keep shoulders
back and straight

keep hips still

POINTS TO WATCH

• Keep your back straight, don't lean forward or arch it, since this will put strain on it.
• Use your abdominals to control the movement; don't lead with your shoulders.
• Keep your hips tucked under and, most importantly, keep them still as you move your chest.

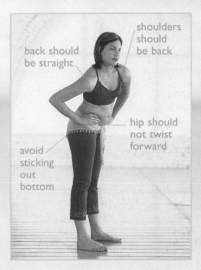

back should
be straight

shoulders
should
be back

avoid
sticking
out
bottom

hip should
not twist
forward

Workout Repetitions	
Beginner	8 times in each direction
Intermediate	24 times in each direction

7 Practice putting steps 2–6 together so that you combine the sliding, lifting, and dropping actions in a smooth, circular movement. *Practice circling in both directions.*

HIP TWIST

Bellydance moves are generally either performed quickly and sharply or more smoothly. This move requires a little of both: The twisting motion is sharp, but the swivel from side to side is soft. It resembles "the twist" dance from the 1950s, although here you don't move your feet from side to side and your chest should remain still. Feel loose and relaxed as you perform this move, since this will help to increase flexibility in the hip area as you twist.

TIPS AND TECHNIQUE
- Try this with up-tempo music, and practice increasing the speed of your twist.
- Keep your chest still as you twist to help define your side abdominals.
- Feel this move in your lower and side abdominals.

keep hips level as you twist

1 Begin in the *Basic Stance* (inset). Keeping your chest still, contract your abdominals and twist your right hip forward as you simultaneously twist your left hip back. Keep your knees soft.

2 Keeping your hips level, contract your abdominals and twist your left hip forward as you simultaneously twist your right hip back. Keep your feet flat on the floor as you twist.

keep hips level

POINTS TO WATCH

• Don't twist your chest and shoulders as you move your hips.
• Keep your hips straight as you twist from side to side.
• Keep your knees soft, and allow them to bend slightly to move your hips, but avoid bending one knee more than the other.

bend knees slightly as you twist

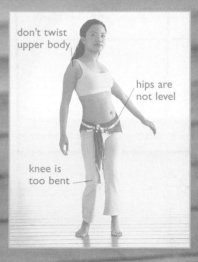

don't twist upper body

hips are not level

knee is too bent

Workout Repetitions	
Beginner	20 times in each direction
Intermediate	40 times in each direction

3 Practice twisting one hip forward, then the other hip, keeping the movement smooth and rhythmic and gradually building up speed.

TUNISIAN TWIST

A fantastic exercise for toning the upper legs, the Tunisian Twist is basically the *Hip Twist* (see pp78–79) performed on one hip. Here you twist your entire leg and hip forward, swivelling on your toes. In the more advanced version of the move, you lift your toes off the floor. This move is typical of the Folk style of bellydance. Position your arms at each side of the twisting hip to draw attention to the movement.

TIPS AND TECHNIQUE

• Target your side abdominals by keeping your chest as still as possible as you twist your hip forward then back.
• Feel this move working your side abdominals and the muscles in your inner thighs and hips.

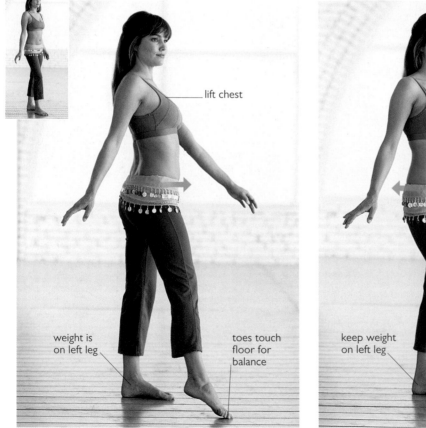

lift chest

weight is on left leg

toes touch floor for balance

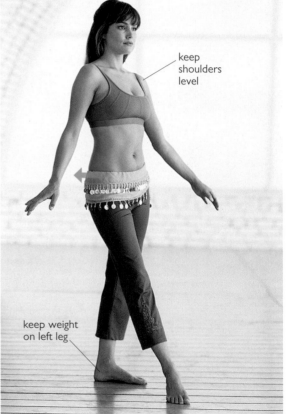

keep shoulders level

keep weight on left leg

1 Stand with your right foot half a step further forward than your left, right knee slightly bent (inset). Contract your abdominals and twist your right hip forward, straightening your leg and raising your heel.

2 Relax your abdominals and twist your right hip back, swivelling on your toes. Remember to keep your chest lifted as you twist.

keep shoulders relaxed

Workout Repetitions	
Beginner	10 times on each side
Intermediate	24 times on each side

don't swing arms

hands are relaxed yet graceful

3 Practice twisting your hip forward then back in a smooth, fluid movement. Try increasing your speed slightly, but be careful to stay rhythmic. *Then practice twisting your left hip forward and back.*

FIGURE EIGHT

This is a sensual movement that opens the hips; as a woman, it should feel very natural and pleasurable to perform it. As you shift your weight, bend your knees slightly to move your hips, but use your abdominals to control the movement and make it smooth and fluid. This move is most effective when performed slowly. Imagine drawing a figure eight with your hips, forming the shape on a flat plain. Try not to lift your hips as you twist them.

TIPS AND TECHNIQUE
• Target your abdominals: Keep your chest still, and make small figure eights.
• Target your hips and thighs: Bend your knees slightly, and make large figure eights.
• Feel this move working your side abdominals, thighs, and hips.

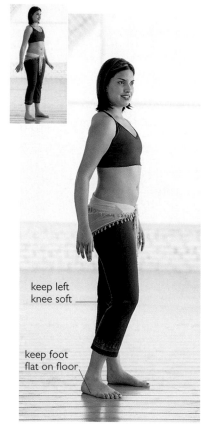

keep left knee soft

keep foot flat on floor

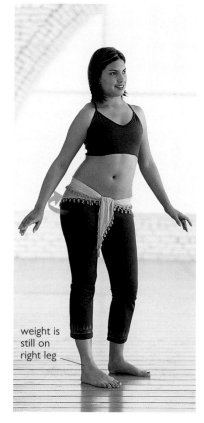

weight is still on right leg

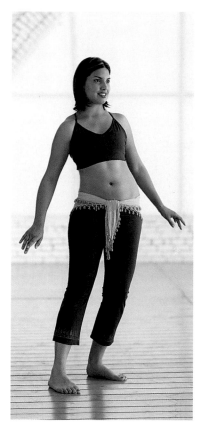

1 Begin in the *Basic Stance* (inset). Twist your right hip forward, bending your right knee and shifting your weight onto your right leg.

2 Contract your abdominals on your right side and twist your right hip back, keeping both knees soft. Be careful not to lock your right leg straight.

3 Push your left hip forward and bend your left knee as you shift your weight onto your left leg.

Workout Repetitions	
Beginner	8 complete Figure Eights
Intermediate	24 complete Figure Eights

relax your arms; allow them to follow your hip movments

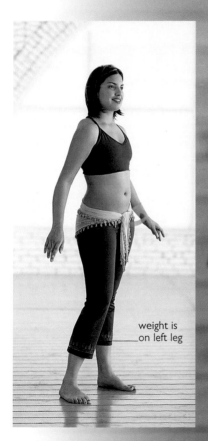

weight is on left leg

4 Complete the Figure Eight by contracting your abdominals on the left side and twisting your left hip back, keeping your knees soft.

5 Practice combining steps 1–4 in a smooth, fluid movement. Be careful to keep your hips level as you shift your weight from side to side.

HIP SNAKE

Move slowly, fluidly, and deliberately when performing the Hip Snake, and note how the knees and foot help to control the vertical circle that the hip makes. Take the undulating movements of the snake as your inspiration when you move your hips. While there are many moves that are fundamental to a bellydancer's repertoire, my students always express joy that they truly "feel" like a bellydancer when they learn this move.

TIPS AND TECHNIQUE
• Make this move more difficult by alternating between right and left Hip Snakes to create a *Figure Eight*-like move in which the eight is vertical.
• Feel this move working your side abdominals and the muscles in your inner thighs and hips.

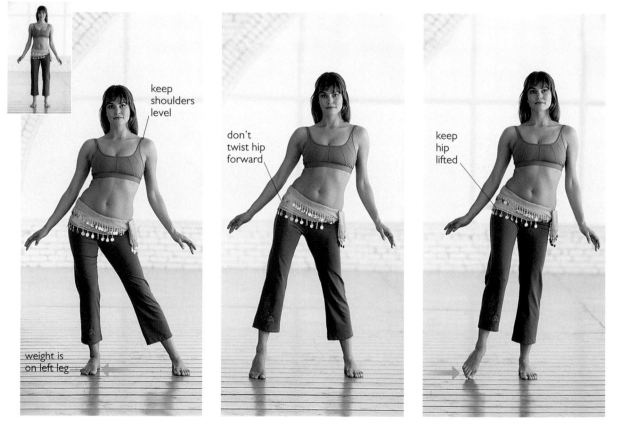

keep shoulders level

weight is on left leg

don't twist hip forward

keep hip lifted

1 Stand in the **Basic Stance** (inset). Step out double hip-width with your right foot, bend your right knee slightly, and push your right hip out to the side.

2 Lift your right heel, and lift your right hip by contracting your side abdominals and straightening your leg. Keep your chest lifted and still.

3 With just the toes touching the floor, slide your right foot in so it is hip-distance from the left. Contract your side abdominals to keep your chest still.

Workout Repetitions	
Beginner	6 times on each side
Intermediate	12 times on each side

keep hands graceful and relaxed

keep knee soft

4 Drop your hip by bending your right leg and relaxing your side abdominals, but remember to keep the toes of your right foot pointed and your heel lifted.

5 Repeat steps 1–4, combining them in a smooth, flowing movement. *Then practice the Hip Snake on the left side.*

MAYA

Here, you reverse the movements of the *Hip Snake* (see pp84–85):
You lift your hip, step out to the side, drop your hip, then slide
your foot back in. The Maya is slightly more challenging—I notice
that many students will begin performing the Maya correctly, then
unknowingly slip into the Hip Snake when they look away from
the mirror. Perform this move slowly, being careful to keep your
hip lifted as you step out to the side.

TIPS AND TECHNIQUE

• For a more sensual effect,
slow the pace as you perform
steps 2 and 3. This also
stretches the side abdominals
more effectively.

• Feel this move in your side
abdominals and the muscles
in your inner thighs and hips.

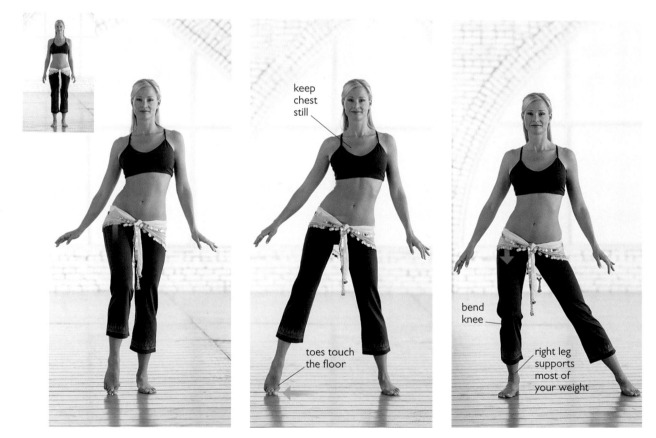

keep
chest
still

toes touch
the floor

bend
knee

right leg
supports
most of
your weight

1 Begin in the *Basic Stance* (inset).
Shift your weight onto your left
leg. Lift your right heel, bend your
right knee, and contract your side
abdominals to raise your right hip.

2 Keeping your hip lifted, with
your right foot, step out to
the right double hip-width as
you straighten your leg. Keep
your heel lifted.

3 Lower your heel so that
your right foot is flat on
the floor, bend your right leg,
and relax your side abdominals
to release your hip.

Workout Repetitions	
Beginner	6 times on each side
Intermediate	12 times on each side

keep your shoulders straight

4 Complete the Maya by smoothly sliding your right foot in to meet your left.

5 Practice combining steps 1–4 into a smooth, controlled, fluid movement. *Then practice the Maya on the left side.*

HIP CAMEL

This sensual hip undulation demonstrates one of the movement principals that make bellydance so unique: As you rock your weight forward and tilt your pelvis down, you actually push out your lower abdominals. Remember to keep your chest lifted and not to allow your shoulders to roll forward. Hip Camels are an excellent way to tone the abdominals without putting stress on the neck or back. Keep the movement slow and fluid.

TIPS AND TECHNIQUE
• Put your hands on your hips to help you feel your pelvis move.
• Push your abdominals out as you tilt your pelvis down, contract them as you tilt your pelvis up.
• Feel this move in your lower abdominals and thighs (quads).

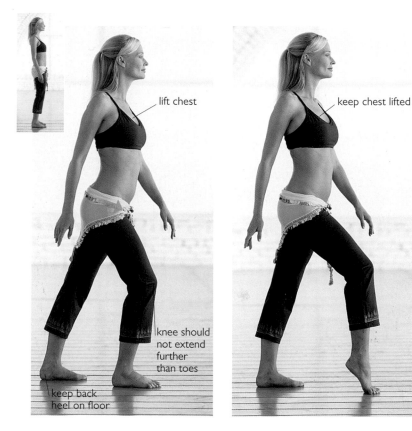

lift chest

keep chest lifted

knee should not extend further than toes

keep back heel on floor

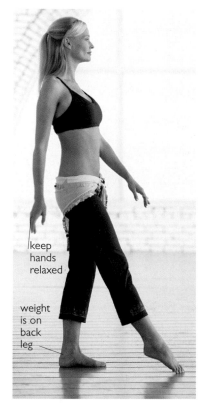

keep hands relaxed

weight is on back leg

1 Begin in the *Basic Stance* (inset). Step forward with your right foot, shifting your weight forward as you bend your right knee, tilt your pelvis down, and push out your lower abdominals.

2 Raise your right heel as you begin contracting your lower abdominals. Use your thighs to control the movement and keep it smooth.

3 Straighten your right leg, and shift your weight back onto your left leg as you tilt your pelvis up and fully contract your abdominals. Keep the toes of your right foot on the floor for balance.

Workout Repetitions	
Beginner	8 times on each leg
Intermediate	16 times on each leg

POINTS TO WATCH

• Don't push your chest forward or pull your shoulders back to exaggerate the undulation, since this will put strain on your lower back.

• Keep your back straight, and generate the movement from your abdominals.

• Keep both feet flat. You are pushing your pelvis too far forward if your back heel lifts off the floor.

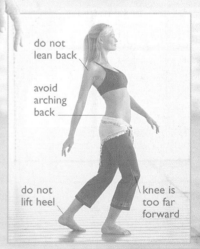

do not lean back

avoid arching back

do not lift heel

knee is too far forward

4 Practice combining steps 1–3, tilting your hips down as you shift your weight forward, then up again as you shift your weight back. The movement should be smooth and undulating. *Then practice the Hip Camel with the left leg forward.*

toes touch floor for balance

TRAVELING SNAKE ARMS

In this, the first of the traveling moves that you'll learn, you combine *Snake Arms* (see pp36–37) with taking small steps forward. If you find the coordination challenging, begin by practicing the feet separately, then add the arms and try counting each step out loud as you perform it. When you begin to link basic moves together into actual sequences, being able to travel adds dimension and dramatic effect to your dance routine.

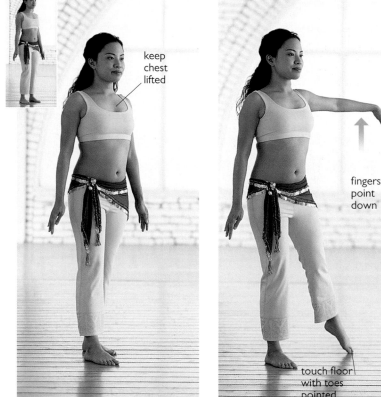

keep chest lifted

fingers point down

touch floor with toes pointed

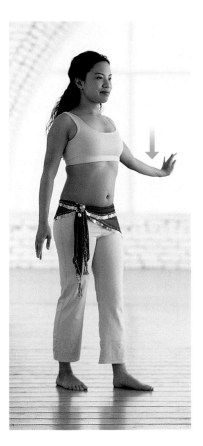

1 Begin in the *Basic Stance* (inset). With your arms at your sides, step forward with your right foot, placing it flat on the floor. Be sure to keep your knees soft.

2 Touch the toes of your left foot out to the left so that your feet are level. Simultaneously raise your left arm (shoulder, elbow, then wrist) to shoulder height at your side.

3 Step forward with your left foot, placing it flat on the floor, as you gracefully lower your left arm, shoulder first, then elbow and wrist.

palm faces
out as arm
is lowered

relax fingers
and keep
hands graceful

5 Step forward with your right foot, placing it flat on the floor, as you gracefully lower your right arm. *Repeat steps 2–5 as necessary to move forward. To finish traveling gracefully, at the end of the final step, step forward with your left foot so that your feet are parallel, and bring your arms down to your sides.*

4 Touch the toes of your right foot out to the right so that your feet are level. As you do this, gracefully raise your right arm (shoulder, elbow, then wrist) to shoulder height at your side.

TRAVELING HIP LIFT AND DROP

Here you combine the *Hip Lift and Drop* (see pp44–45) with walking forward. Put the accent on the lift, making the movement as sharp and dramatic as possible—wearing a coin- or bead-fringed hip scarf will help you to hear this. Take small, manageable steps to make it easier to balance and maintain rhythm. This is an excellent traveling step to dance when you want to make an entrance. The higher you lift your hip, the more seductive the move will look.

TIPS AND TECHNIQUE

• Try combining this move with *Goddess Arms*: Place your hand on your hip as you lift it, then alternate hand positions as you step forward and lift the other hip,
• Feel this move working the fronts of your thighs and your side and lower abdominals.

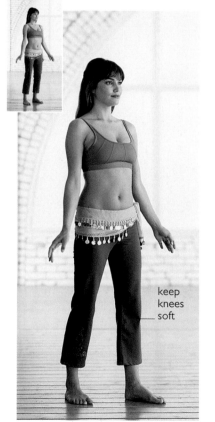

keep knees soft

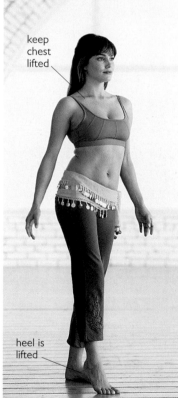

keep chest lifted

heel is lifted

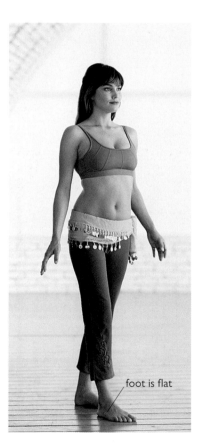

foot is flat

1 Begin in the *Basic Stance* (inset). Step forward with your left foot, placing it flat on the floor in front of you. Be sure to keep your chest lifted.

2 Step forward with your right foot, touching the floor with your toes as you contract your side abdominals and lift your right hip without twisting it forward.

3 Step forward with your right foot, placing it flat on the floor in front of you, as you release your side abdominals and drop your hip.

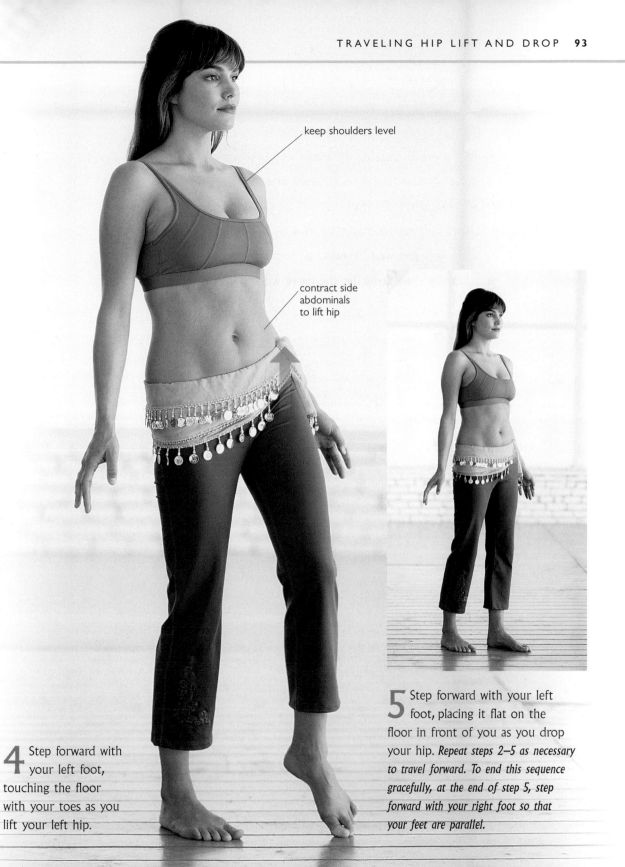

keep shoulders level

contract side
abdominals
to lift hip

4 Step forward with
your left foot,
touching the floor
with your toes as you
lift your left hip.

5 Step forward with your left
foot, placing it flat on the
floor in front of you as you drop
your hip. *Repeat steps 2–5 as necessary
to travel forward. To end this sequence
gracefully, at the end of step 5, step
forward with your right foot so that
your feet are parallel.*

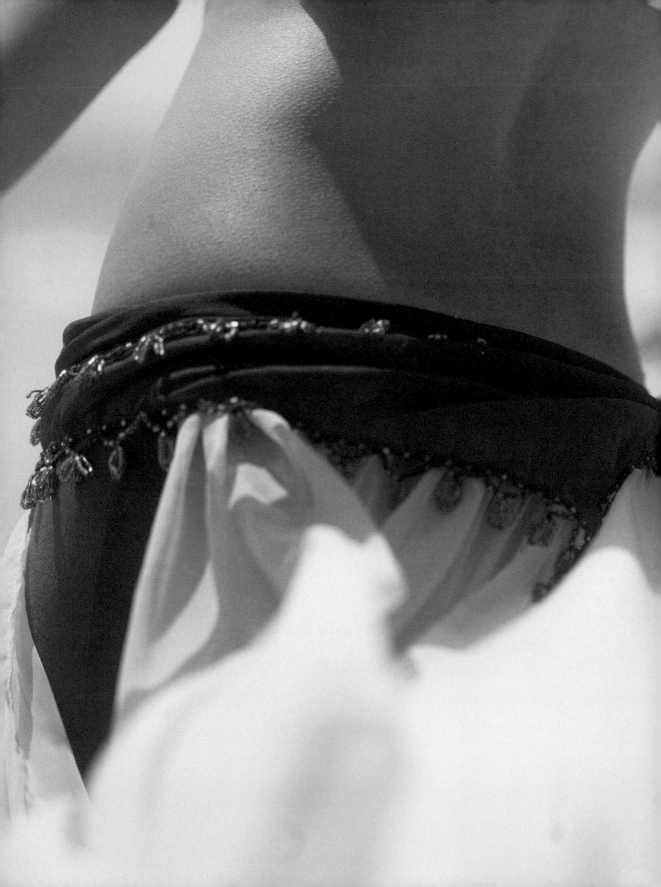

DANCE ROUTINE

LEVEL TWO

This dance sequence links together movements learned in *Basic Moves Level Two*. This is where you learn to add dimension to a dance by incorporating traveling moves. Let your arm and hand movements be graceful and flowing, but remember to keep your neck and shoulders relaxed and your chest lifted. Once again, the sequence is presented in three parts, each consisting of an eight-count sequence. Counting out loud as you perform each step will help you to keep your rhythm.

GODDESS DANCE, PART ONE

In this routine, you learn to incorporate traveling moves into the dance sequence. You may want to practice just the footwork to begin with. When you have learned the routine, begin adding some expression. Perform the *Traveling Hip Lifts* with attitude, and try turning your head in the direction of your arms as you undulate them for *Traveling Snake Arms*.

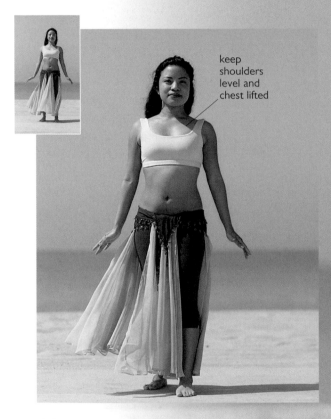

keep shoulders level and chest lifted

1 Start in the **Basic Stance** (inset). Begin a *Traveling Hip Lift* on the right side by stepping forward with your left foot, placing it flat in front of you.

2 Touch the toes of your right foot forward as you sharply lift your right hip. As you do this, move your arms into *Goddess Arms* pose with your right hand on your hip to emphasize the lift, and your left hand just behind your head.

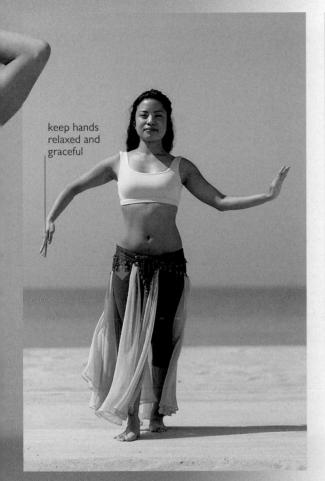

keep hands
relaxed and
graceful

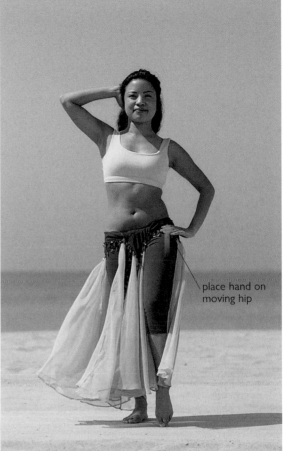

place hand on
moving hip

3 Complete the *Traveling Hip Lift* on the right side by stepping forward flat with your right foot as you release your right hip. Begin alternating your arm position, moving your left hand toward your left hip and your right hand toward your head.

4 Begin a *Traveling Hip Lift* on the left side by touching the toes of your left foot forward as you sharply lift your left hip. As you do this, move your arms into *Goddess Arms* with your left hand on your hip and your right hand behind your head.

▶

At a glance

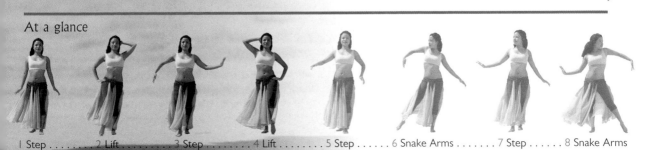

I Step . . . . 2 Lift . . . . 3 Step . . . . 4 Lift . . . . 5 Step . . . . . . 6 Snake Arms . . . . 7 Step . . . . . 8 Snake Arms

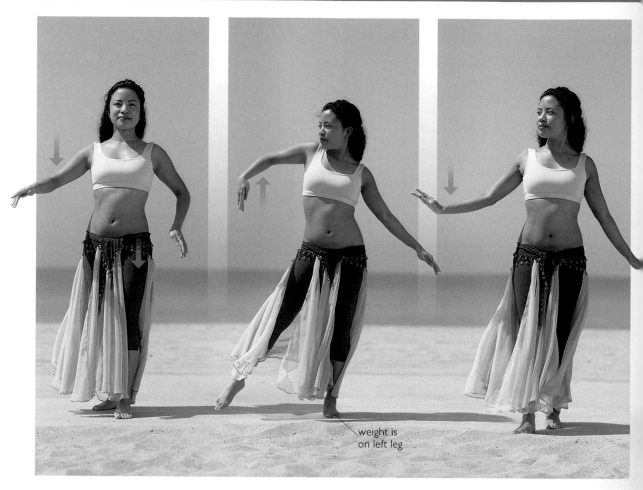

weight is
on left leg

5 Step forward flat with your left foot as you release your left hip. Begin elegantly lowering your right arm to your side in preparation for *Traveling Snake Arms* on the right side.

6 Touch the toes of your right foot out to the right as you raise your right arm (shoulder, elbow, then wrist) and perform a graceful *Traveling Snake Arm* on the right side.

7 Step forward flat with your right foot as you gracefully lower your right arm in the same order that you raised it. Incorporate poise and elegance into your moves.

At a glance

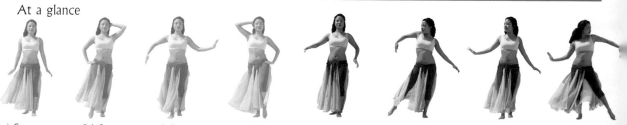

I Step . . . . 2 Lift . . . . 3 Step . . . . 4 Lift . . . . 5 Step . . . . . . 6 Snake Arms . . . . 7 Step . . . . . . 8 Snake Arms

turn head in
direction of
raised arm

raise arm with
palm of hand
facing inward

8 Touch the toes of your left foot out to the left as you perform a *Traveling Snake Arm* by raising your left arm and lowering your right. Finish this sequence with your left leg extended to the left, toes pointed and touching the ground, and your left arm extended at your side.

GODDESS DANCE, PART TWO

Although you step out to the side and then forward in this sequence, you don't actually travel. The key to making this part of the dance appear easy and fluid is to be aware of your center of balance and to focus on shifting your weight effectively. Convey pride and sensuality as you dance. Count the eight beats as you move to help you keep your rhythm.

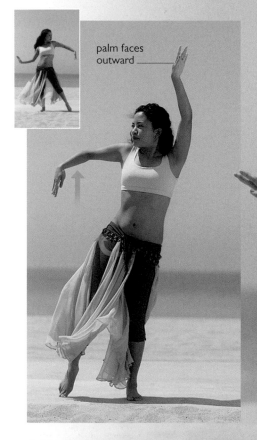

palm faces outward

keep chest lifted

1 Move from *Traveling Snake Arms* with your left arm (inset), and begin a *Hip Snake* with your right hip: Shift your weight onto your left leg and smoothly push your right hip out and up. As you do this, extend your left arm above your head and perform *Isis Arms* with your right arm, raising your shoulder, elbow, then wrist.

2 Complete the *Hip Snake* on the right side by sliding your right foot in and smoothly releasing your right hip. Simultaneously lower your right arm.

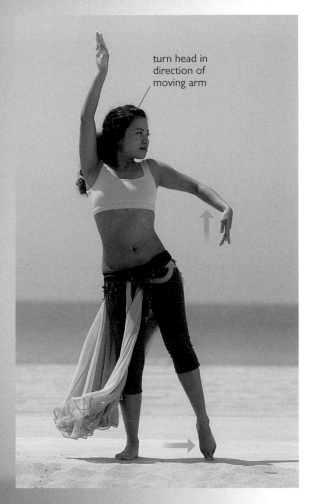

turn head in direction of moving arm

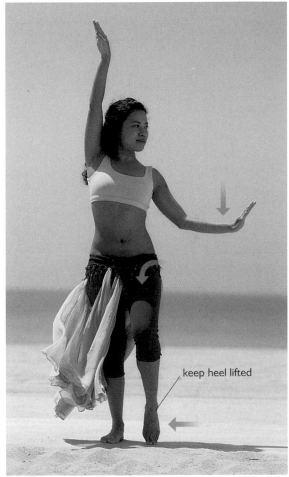

keep heel lifted

3 Begin a *Hip Snake* on the left side by shifting your weight onto your right leg and stepping out to the left with your left foot, toes pointed, as you push your left hip out and up. As you do this, perform *Isis Arms*, this time raising your left arm.

4 Complete the *Hip Snake* on the left side by sliding your left foot in, toes still pointed, and smoothly releasing your hip. As you do this, gracefully complete *Isis Arms* by lowering your left arm: Shoulder first, then elbow and wrist.

At a glance

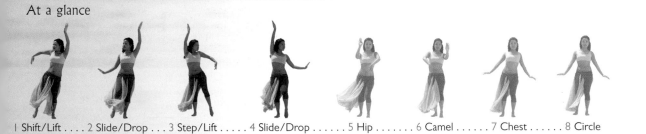

1 Shift/Lift . . . . 2 Slide/Drop . . . 3 Step/Lift . . . . . 4 Slide/Drop . . . . . . 5 Hip . . . . 6 Camel . . . . . . 7 Chest . . . . . . 8 Circle

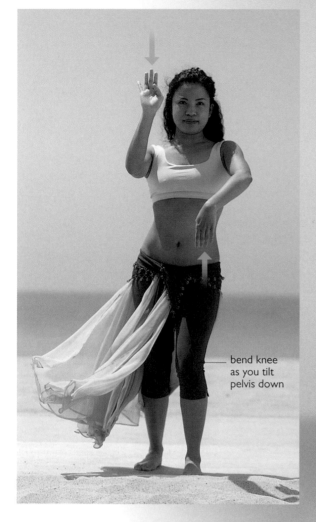

bend knee
as you tilt
pelvis down

straighten
as you tilt
pelvis up

5 Perform the first half of a *Hip Camel* by stepping forward with your left foot and shifting your weight forward as you tilt your pelvis down. As you do this, begin performing *Mermaid Arms* by gracefully raising your left arm in front of you as you lower your right arm.

6 Complete the *Hip Camel* by shifting your weight back as you tilt your pelvis up. Continue to perform *Mermaid Arms,* gracefully raising your right arm in front of you as you lower your left.

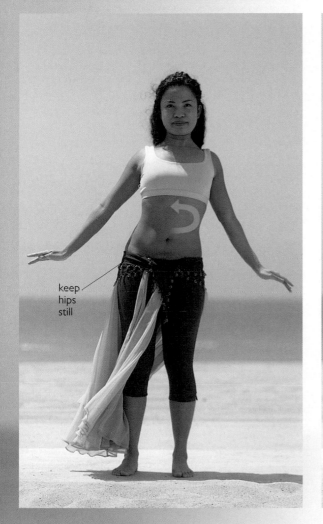

keep hips still

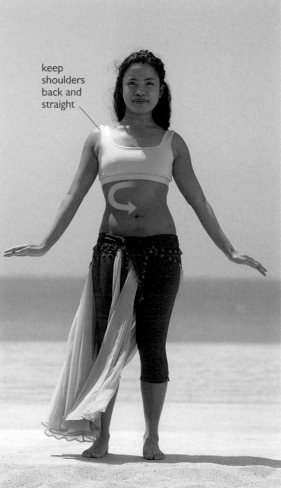

keep shoulders back and straight

7 Move your arms to your sides, and step your left foot back so that your feet are parallel and hip-width apart. Begin a *Chest Circle* by lengthening your abdominals and sliding your ribcage to the left, then up.

8 Keeping the movement as smooth as possible and isolating it to the upper body, complete the *Chest Circle* by sliding your ribcage to the right, then down and back to the center.

At a glance

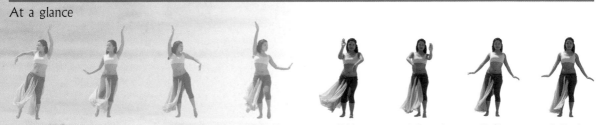

I Shift/Lift . . . . 2 Slide/Drop . . . 3 Step/Lift . . . . . 4 Slide/Drop . . . . . . 5 Hip . . . . 6 Camel . . . . . . 7 Chest . . . . . 8 Circle

GODDESS DANCE FINALE

In Basic Moves Level Two, you learned the *Maya* and the *Figure Eight* both broken down into four steps each, but in this sequence you perform each move over two beats. When performing the *Tunisian Twist*, be careful not to lift your hip. Holding your hands at your sides draws attention to and "frames" your hip movements.

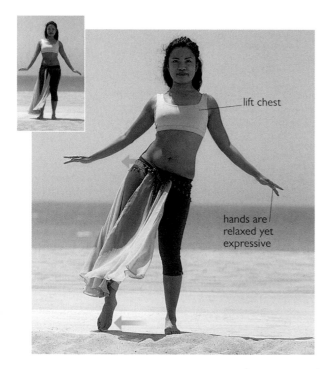

lift chest

hands are relaxed yet expressive

keep shoulders level

1 Move from the *Chest Circle* (inset), and perform a *Maya* on the right side by shifting your weight onto your left leg, smoothly lifting your right hip, and touching the toes of your right foot out to the right. Keep your arms extended low at your sides.

2 Complete the *Maya* on the right side by dropping your hip and sliding your right foot in so it is hip-distance from the left, toes still pointed. Be sure to keep your shoulders back and level. Your weight is on your left leg.

At a glance

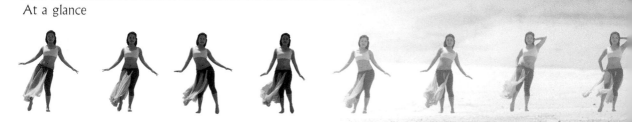

⌐ Lift/Step . . . . . 2 Drop/Slide . . . . 3 Lift/Step . . . .4 Drop/Slide . . . . 5 Figure Eight . . . 6 Figure Eight . . . 7 Twist Forward . . . 8 Twist B.

relax shoulders and neck

keep abdominals tucked in

3 Shift your weight onto your right leg, and begin a *Maya* on the left side by smoothly lifting your left hip and touching the toes of your left foot out to the left.

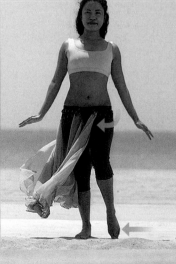

4 Complete the *Maya* on the left side by dropping your left hip and sliding your left foot in so it is hip-distance from the right, toes still pointed.

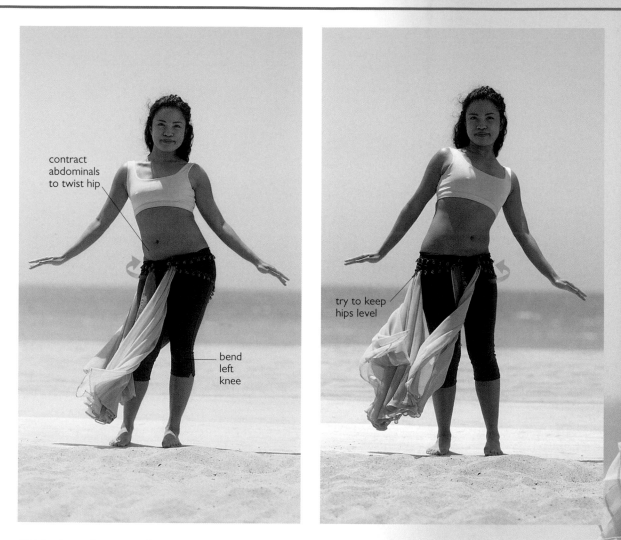

contract
abdominals
to twist hip

bend
left
knee

try to keep
hips level

5 Begin performing a *Figure Eight,* starting on the right side, by shifting your weight to your right leg, bending your right knee, and smoothly twisting your right hip back.

6 Shift your weight onto your left leg and complete the *Figure Eight* by bending your left knee and smoothly twisting your left hip back. Be sure to keep your chest lifted.

At a glance

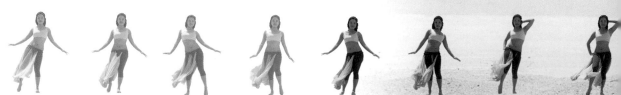

1 Lift/Step . . . . . 2 Drop/Slide . . . . 3 Lift/Step . . . .4 Drop/Slide . . . . 5 Figure Eight . . . 6 Figure Eight . . . 7 Twist Forward . . . 8 Twist B

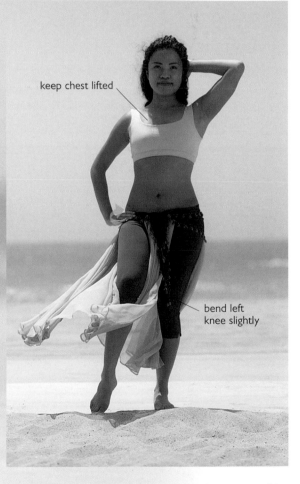

keep chest lifted

bend left
knee slightly

7 With weight on your left leg, touch the toes of your right foot forward, and begin a *Tunisian Twist* by smoothly twisting your right hip forward. As you do this, put your right hand on your hip and your left behind your head in *Goddess Arms.*

8 Finish the sequence by sharply twisting your hip back, your right foot still on its toes. Bend your left knee slightly, lift your chest, and look forward proudly to end the sequence.

GODDESS DANCE SUMMARY

Use this summary for quick reference when performing the entire Goddess Dance, or even different parts of it. Flow rhythmically from one step to the next, adding expression to make the dance your own. Moves on the right side are indicated with an "R" and moves on the left with an "L."

Goddess Dance, Part One

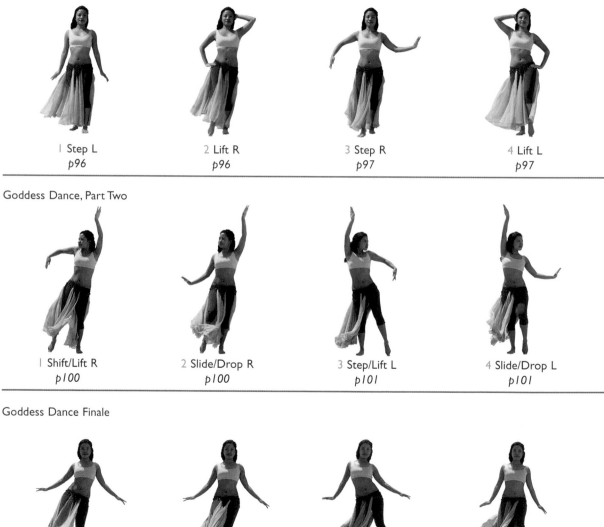

1 Step L	2 Lift R	3 Step R	4 Lift L
p96	p96	p97	p97

Goddess Dance, Part Two

1 Shift/Lift R	2 Slide/Drop R	3 Step/Lift L	4 Slide/Drop L
p100	p100	p101	p101

Goddess Dance Finale

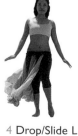

1 Lift/Step R	2 Drop/Slide R	3 Lift/Step L	4 Drop/Slide L
p104	p104	p105	p105

*Enjoy letting go. Dancing can be
a journey of self-discovery.*

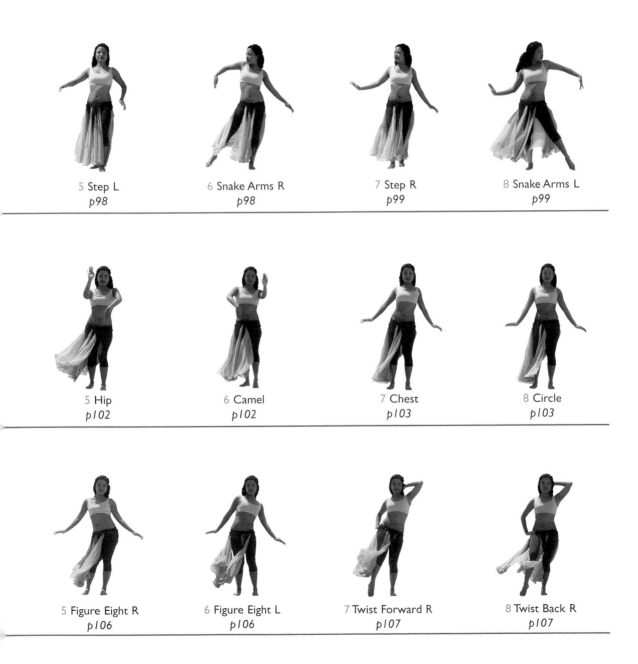

5 Step L	6 Snake Arms R	7 Step R	8 Snake Arms L
p98	p98	p99	p99

5 Hip	6 Camel	7 Chest	8 Circle
p102	p102	p103	p103

5 Figure Eight R	6 Figure Eight L	7 Twist Forward R	8 Twist Back R
p106	p106	p107	p107

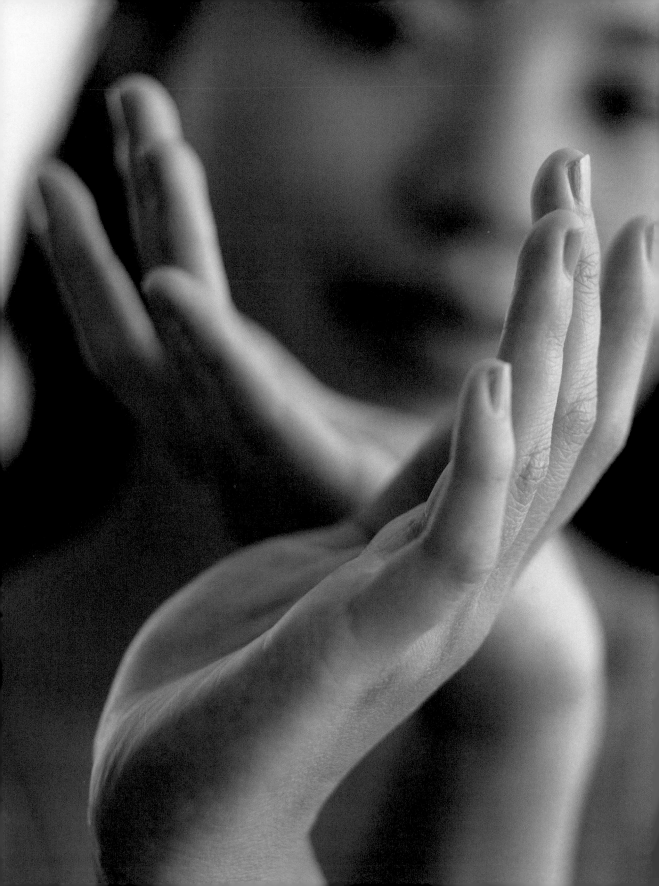

BASIC
MOVES
LEVEL THREE

Building on the skills learned in Basic Moves
Levels One and Two, Level Three introduces
challenging moves that require advanced muscle
control. In the Body Wave, for example, you learn
to isolate the abdominals in order to make a
smooth transition between a hip and a chest
movement. This is where you also learn the
dynamic Four-Count Turn. Don't overlook moves
that appear simple, such as Hand Undulations—
perfecting a graceful flutter of the hand is essential
for conveying expression in your dance.

HEAD SLIDE

This ancient Egyptian-inspired move involves isolating your head and moving it independently of your shoulders. The Head Slide is most often performed with Temple Arms, as demonstrated here. The raised hands allow the arms to frame the sliding movement of the head. You might also try holding a veil taut and peeking seductively over the edge as you slide your head from side to side. If you have tense neck and shoulder muscles, you may find this challenging.

TIPS AND TECHNIQUE

• Practice steps 5–8 of the *Goddess Salutation* to help increase flexibility in your neck and shoulder muscles.
• Feel this move in your neck muscles; it lengthens and strengthens them and helps to relieve tension.

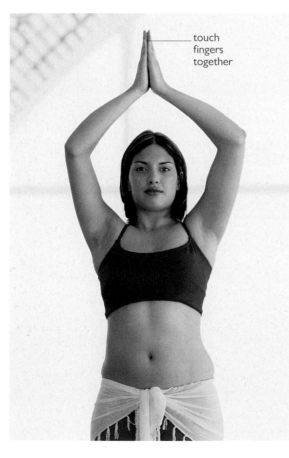

touch fingers together

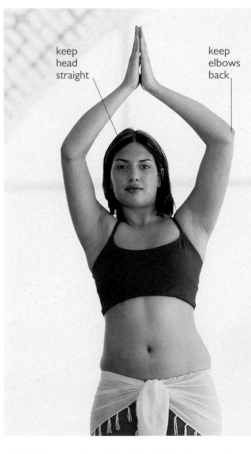

keep head straight

keep elbows back

1 Position your arms in Temple Arms with hands together above your head, palms facing, fingers pointing upward, and elbows out to the sides. Align your hands over the center of your head.

2 Slide your head to the right, keeping it as straight as you can. Be sure to keep your shoulders relaxed. Try not to allow your body to lean to the right.

relax your hands—don't
press them together

relax your arms

stand up straight
with chest lifted

POINTS TO WATCH

• Keep your head straight as
you slide it to the side; don't
reach with your chin.
• Ensure that your elbows and
hands don't drop forward or
fall to one side.
• If you find this difficult to
begin with, don't let it show.
Avoid straining your face and
tensing your facial muscles.

3 Slide your head
to the left,
remembering to keep
your head straight so
that your ears are level.
Repeat, sliding your
head from side to side.

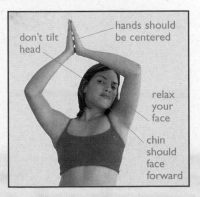

don't tilt
head

hands should
be centered

relax
your
face

chin
should
face
forward

HAND UNDULATIONS

Students new to bellydance will often neglect their hands when they dance, concentrating instead on dramatic hip and belly movements. Your hands are essential for lending expression and grace to your movements; it takes practice to perfect the refined hand movements characteristic of bellydance. In Egypt, many of the best bellydancers attend ballet schools to learn and perfect hand movements alone. Hand Undulations can be performed with a single hand at the side of the body or with both hands at chest or face level (see *Butterfly Hands*, opposite). Once you've mastered the movement, try outlining the curves of your body while undulating your hands.

TIPS AND TECHNIQUES
• Relax your hands before you begin: Make a tight fist, then extend your hands fully, stretching your fingers back. Repeat this 5 times.
• Perform Hand Undulations as a flowing complement to *Hip Snakes* or to soften a sharp move such as a *Hip Lift*.

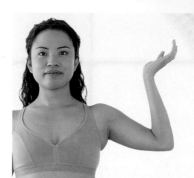

1 Start with your hand positioned level with your head, palm facing up, and elbow out to your side.

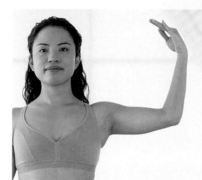

2 Lift your hand so that your palm faces you. Keep your hand relaxed and fingers graceful.

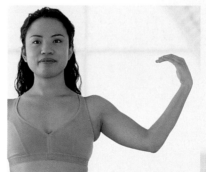

3 Begin curling your fingers away from you, pulling them back slightly.

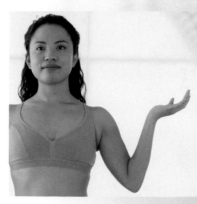

4 Curl your fingers back entirely and finish with your palm facing upward.

keep fingers
slightly separated
and graceful _____

5 Combine steps 1–4 and
practice undulating your
hand, moving it between head and
shoulder level. *Practice this with one
hand, then with the other.*

BUTTERFLY HANDS

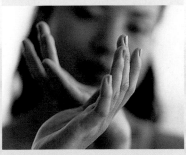

Try this seductive variation of
Hand Undulations. Practice
undulating both hands, this time
in front of you at face level. Peek
through your moving hands as you
alternately hold both palms face
up, then turn them both downward.

SHOULDER SHIMMY

The shoulders and neck are notoriously tense—we hold much of our stress in this area of the body—so loosening some of this muscle stiffness before you begin will help you to master this move more effectively (*see right*). Start slowly and gradually build up speed until your shimmy becomes more of a vibration. This is a deceptively challenging move, but have fun with it and focus on maintaining your rhythm to help keep your shimmy going.

TIPS AND TECHNIQUE
- Relax your shoulders before you begin by circling each shoulder forward 5 times.
- Try traveling with the Shoulder Shimmy by taking small steps forward.
- Feel this move in your shoulders, upper back, upper abdominals, chest, and upper arms.

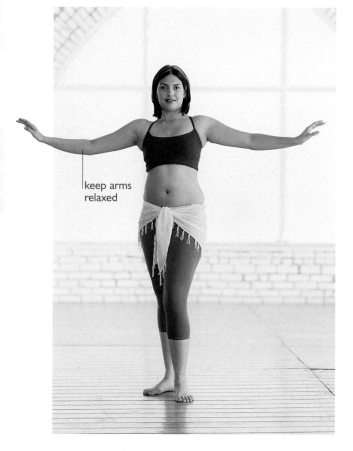

keep arms relaxed

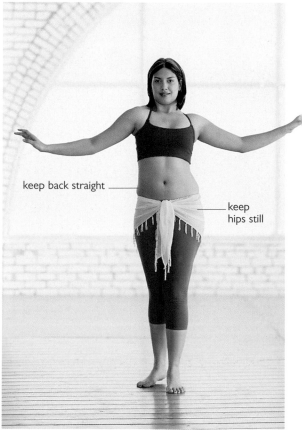

keep back straight

keep hips still

1 Stand with one foot slightly further forward than the other and extend your arms at shoulder height at your sides. Keep your shoulders down, your neck relaxed, and your back straight.

2 Push your right shoulder forward, being careful to keep your neck relaxed. Keep your hips as still as possible to help focus attention on your shoulders.

lead movement with
your shoulders

hands are relaxed
and graceful

4 Practice pushing each
shoulder forward then
back, gradually speeding the
movement up into a rhythmic
shimmy. The faster you shimmy,
the less distance your shoulders
move back and forth.

3 Push your left shoulder forward as you
pull your right shoulder back. Keep your
arms relaxed at your sides—don't allow them
to move about too much.

Workout Repetitions	
Beginner	10 seconds
Intermediate	25 seconds

CHEST CAMEL

Like the *Hip Camel* (see pp88–89), the Chest Camel tones the abdominals without putting strain on the neck or back. The most common mistake when learning this move is to swoop forward, leading with the head and shoulders and over-arching the back. Use your upper abdominals to control the movement. Performed correctly, the Chest Camel looks fluid and quite mesmerizing. Because it strengthens the abdominals, this move can help to improve your posture.

TIPS AND TECHNIQUE
• Make this move more challenging by practicing it with your hands by your sides instead of on your hips.
• Feel this move lengthening your upper abdominals as well as working the upper back and chest muscles.

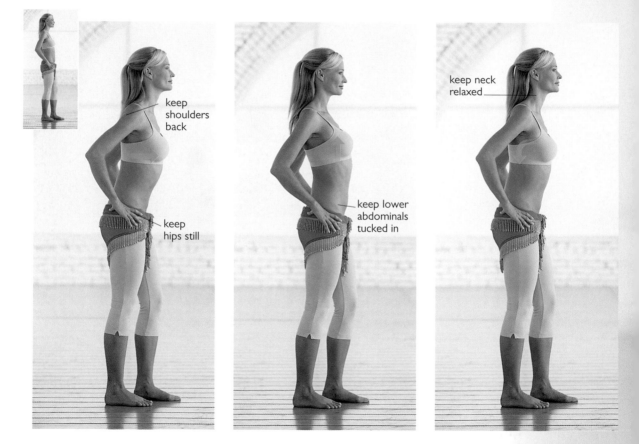

keep shoulders back

keep hips still

keep lower abdominals tucked in

keep neck relaxed

1 Stand with hands on your hips, one foot slightly forward to keep you steady (inset). Lengthen your upper abdominals and push your chest forward.

2 Lengthen your abdominals further and lift your chest. Be careful not to arch your back too much and not to allow your lower body and hips to move.

3 Pull your chest back slightly and drop it by contracting your upper abdominals, keeping the movement slow and controlled. Avoid tilting your hips forward.

Workout Repetitions	
Beginner	6 times
Intermediate	18 times

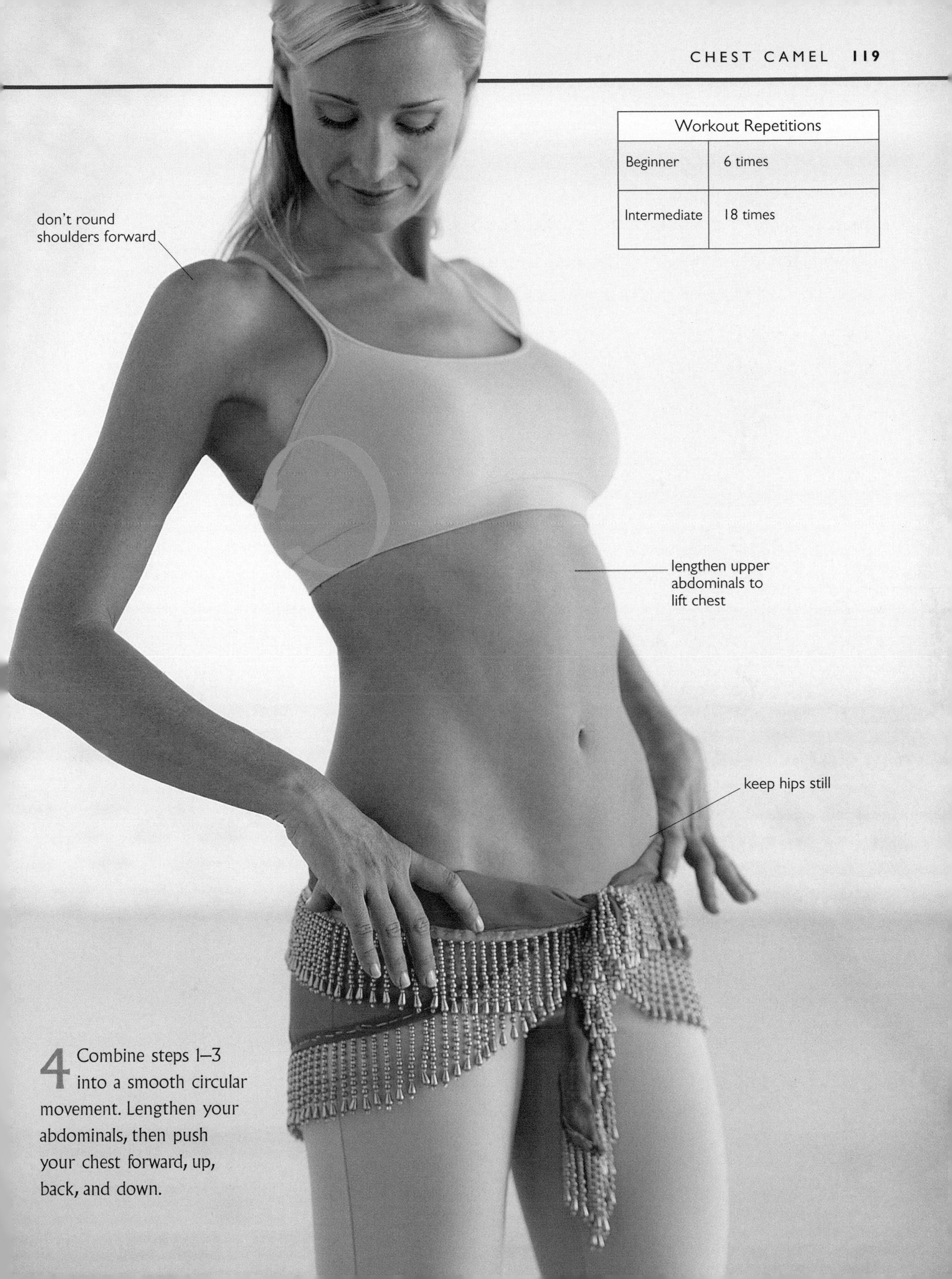

don't round
shoulders forward

lengthen upper
abdominals to
lift chest

keep hips still

4 Combine steps 1–3
into a smooth circular
movement. Lengthen your
abdominals, then push
your chest forward, up,
back, and down.

BODY WAVE

This is one of my favorite moves, but it is also one of the most challenging. It combines the movements of the *Hip Camel* (see pp88–89) and the *Chest Camel* (see pp116–117) in a dramatic full-body undulation that is guaranteed to impress. Use abdominal control to make a smooth transition between the hip and chest movements. To make your movements rhythmic, count steps one and three as you perform them (but not two, since it is the transition).

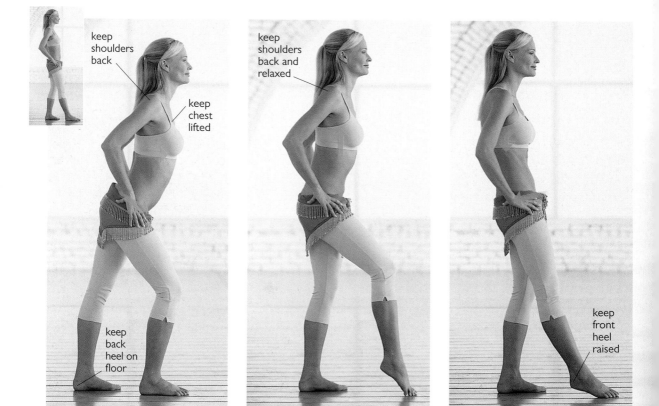

keep shoulders back

keep chest lifted

keep back heel on floor

keep shoulders back and relaxed

keep front heel raised

1 Stand with right foot forward, hands on hips (inset). Shift your weight onto your right leg, bending it slightly as you tilt your hips down and lengthen your upper abdominals to push your chest forward.

2 Continue lengthening your abdominals to lift your chest as you simultaneously bring your right heel off the floor. Use your right thigh to keep you steady.

3 Pull your chest back, smoothly dropping it down as you shift your weight back onto your left leg, tilt your hips up, and straighten your right leg. Keep the movement slow and conrolled.

Workout Repetitions	
Beginner	6 times on each leg
Intermediate	12 times on each leg

relax neck and shoulders

keep chest lifted

POINTS TO WATCH

• Keep your neck and shoulders relaxed and your chin slightly lifted. Your shoulders move with your chest but don't lead the movement.
• Avoid lifting your back heel off the floor as you push your chest forward; this means you are using your legs, not your abdominals, to control the movement.

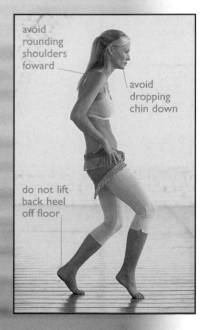

avoid rounding shoulders foward

avoid dropping chin down

do not lift back heel off floor

4 Repeat steps 1–3, keeping the movement as fluid as possible. *Then practice the move with your left leg forward.*

TRAVELING HIP SNAKE

In this move you combine the undulations of the *Hip Snake* (see pp84–85) with stepping to the side. This is the only traveling step where you move to the side, which makes it very useful when you begin linking moves together in sequences, since it adds another dimension to your dance. Here you travel to the left, and what you may find difficult initially is that you raise the opposite, right hip. Allow your arms to follow the movements of your hip.

TIPS AND TECHNIQUE
• Adjust the size of your steps to fit your dance area.
• Master this move by practicing just the footwork to begin with, then adding the hip undulation.
• Feel this move in your side abdominals as well as the muscles in your thighs and hips.

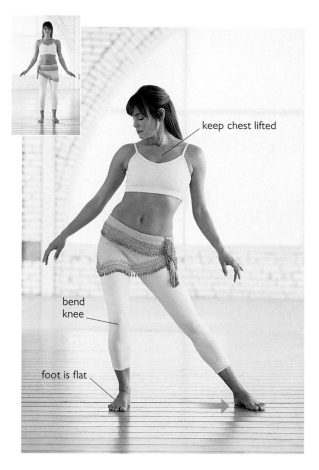

keep chest lifted

bend knee

foot is flat

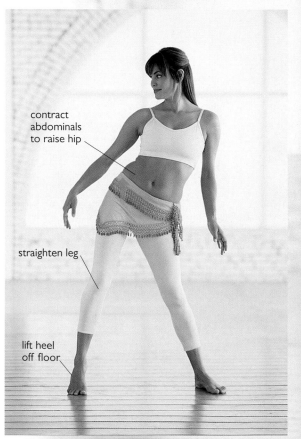

contract abdominals to raise hip

straighten leg

lift heel off floor

1 Begin in the *Basic Stance* (inset). Step out double hip-width to the left as you bend your right knee, shift your weight onto your right leg, and push your right hip out to the side.

2 Bring your right heel off the floor as you straighten your right leg and contract your side abdominals to raise your right hip. Take care to keep your shoulders level.

keep chest lifted and
shoulders level

shoulders
are level

weight is
on left leg

keep heel
lifted as you
slide foot in

3 Shift your weight
onto your left leg
and slide your right foot
in to meet your left,
keeping your heel
and hip lifted.

4 Release your side abdominals,
dropping your hip and bending
your right knee slightly as you lower
your right heel. *Repeat steps 1–4 to
continue to travel to the left. Reverse
the steps to travel to the right.*

TRAVELING HIP CAMEL

To travel while performing a *Hip Camel* (see pp88–89), step forward as you tilt your hips down and push out your abdominals. Then tilt your hips up and contract your abdominals as you begin to take your next step. The most common mistake students make when learning this move is to put too much emphasis on the feet and to kick up when stepping. Isolate your hips, and be careful not to rock your body forward as you step.

TIPS AND TECHNIQUE
• Take smaller steps to make it easier to keep your rhythm.
• Tone and firm your buns by taking larger steps and squeezing your buns in step 2.
• Feel this move working your lower abdominals and the fronts of your thighs.

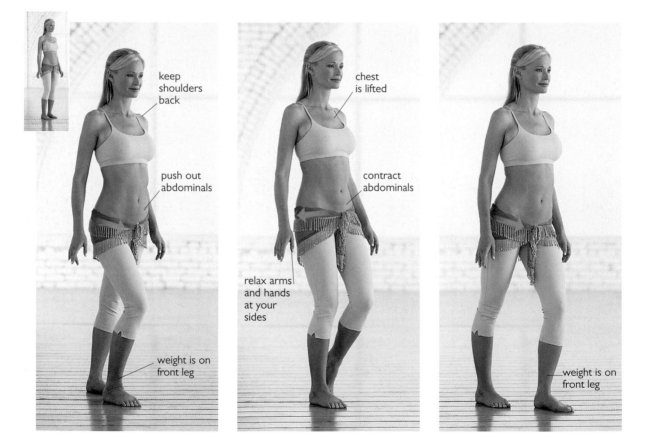

keep shoulders back

push out abdominals

weight is on front leg

chest is lifted

contract abdominals

relax arms and hands at your sides

weight is on front leg

1 Begin in the *Basic Stance* (inset). Step forward with your right foot, shifting your weight forward as you bend your knee, tilt your hips down, and push out your abdominals.

2 Contract your abdominals, and start to tilt your hips up as you begin stepping forward with your left foot. Be careful to keep your chest lifted.

3 Step down flat with your left foot, and shift your weight forward as you bend your left knee, tilt your hips down, and push out your abdominals.

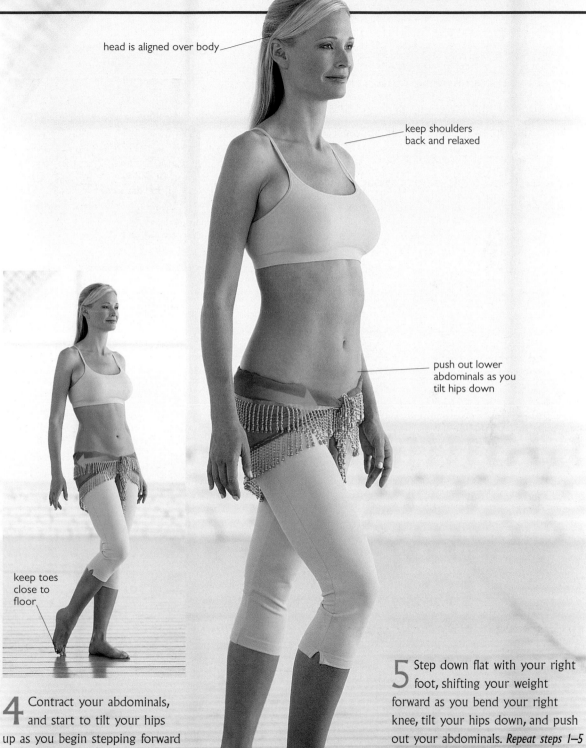

head is aligned over body

keep shoulders back and relaxed

push out lower abdominals as you tilt hips down

keep toes close to floor

4 Contract your abdominals, and start to tilt your hips up as you begin stepping forward with your right foot. Be careful not to lean back.

5 Step down flat with your right foot, shifting your weight forward as you bend your right knee, tilt your hips down, and push out your abdominals. *Repeat steps 1–5 to travel forward. To end the sequence gracefully, step your feet together.*

TRAVELING HIP TWIST

When you twist your right hip forward, your left hip automatically twists back. Be sure to keep your hips level as you focus on this swiveling action. Remembering that your hips are connected will help you to make this move look smooth and effortless. Wear a coin- or bead-fringed hip scarf, and use the noise that it make as you twist forward and back to help you keep your rhythm. This move is typical of the *ghawazee* Folk-style of bellydance.

TIPS AND TECHNIQUE

• Be careful not to lock your knees straight—bend them slightly when you step, otherwise this move can look very wooden.
• Don't allow your upper body to twist as you move your hips.
• Feel this move working your side abdominals and defining your waist.

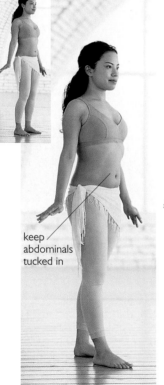

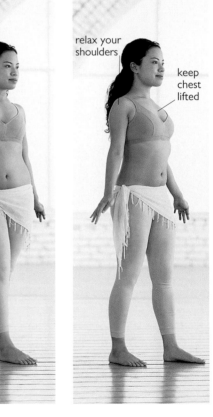

keep abdominals tucked in

keep foot on floor as you twist

keep hips level

relax your shoulders

keep chest lifted

1 Begin in the *Basic Stance* (inset). Step forward flat with your right foot. Be sure to keep your chest lifted.

2 Twist your right hip forward, keeping your right leg straight. Avoid twisting your upper body.

3 Twist your hip back, remembering to keep your hips as level as possible and your knees very slightly bent.

4 Shift your weight onto your right leg and take a small step forward flat with your left foot.

keep chest lifted

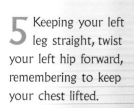
foot stays on floor

5 Keeping your left leg straight, twist your left hip forward, remembering to keep your chest lifted.

6 Twist your hip back. *Repeat steps 1–6 to travel forward. To finish traveling gracefully, at the end of step 6, shift your weight onto your left leg and step forward with your right foot so that your feet are parallel.*

FOUR-COUNT TURN

The turn is broken down into five steps rather than four because it makes it easier to learn the footwork. Run through these steps slowly, then combine steps two and three, the crossing and pivoting, and count four beats as you turn. To begin with, you may find the footwork slightly awkward, but as you speed up, it will come more naturally to you. Perform one turn for dramatic effect or, when you feel confident, try performing several in quick succession.

TIPS AND TECHNIQUE
• When performing successive turns, always pause briefly between each one to avoid dizziness.
• To prevent dizziness when performing successive turns, try "spotting:" Pick a spot in the direction you are turning and focus on it until you complete the turn.

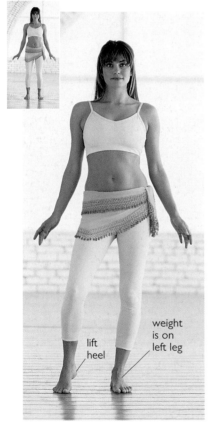

lift heel

weight is on left leg

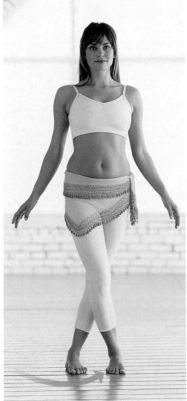

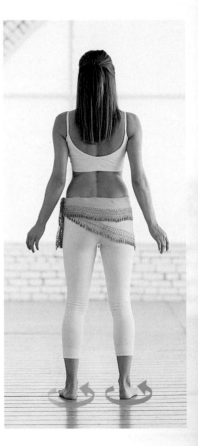

1 Begin in the *Basic Stance* (inset). Shift your weight onto your left leg and lift your right heel slightly. Keep your shoulders relaxed and your chest lifted.

2 Cross your right leg in front of your left. As you step your foot across, notice how your hips follow and begin to turn.

3 Pivot on the balls of your feet, turning 180° to your left. Be careful to keep your chest lifted and your body upright, since this will aid your balance.

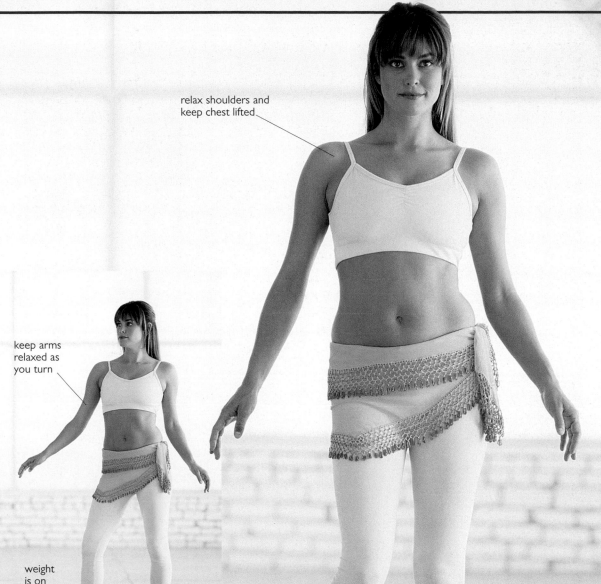

relax shoulders and
keep chest lifted

keep arms
relaxed as
you turn

weight
is on
right leg

4 With your weight on your right
leg, swing your left leg behind you
and turn your body, placing your foot
so it faces forward. Stay relaxed and
enjoy the freedom of the movement.

5 Gracefully slide your
right foot in, bending
your right knee slightly
and assuming a finishing
pose. *Then practice turning
to your right.*

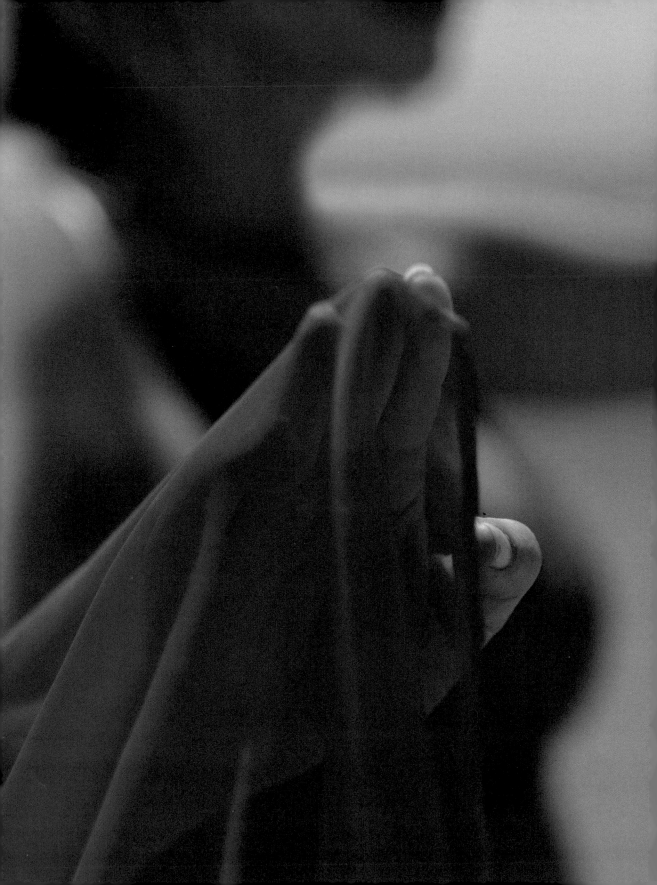

DANCE ROUTINE
LEVEL THREE

In this final dance sequence you link together
moves learned throughout the book, and have the
added challenge of performing them with a veil.
If you don't have a veil, use a shawl made of light-
weight fabric instead. Dancing with a veil helps
you to make your arm movements more graceful
and elegant, but it also enhances your workout.
The Veil Dance is presented in three parts, each
made up of an eight-count sequence.

VEIL DANCE, PART ONE

In this final routine you learn to dance with a veil. You can perform the routine without it, but a veil adds grace and mystique and helps make you more aware of your arm movements. Hold the veil between your first and second fingers, and let it be an extension of your arms, allowing it to trail gently behind you as you move. Start at the back of your dance space—in this part of the routine, you travel forward.

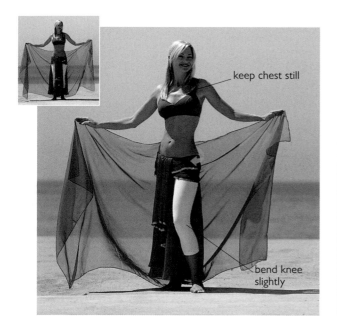

keep chest still

bend knee slightly

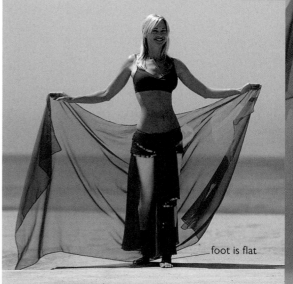

foot is flat

1 Begin in the *Basic Stance*. Hold your veil behind you with arms slightly raised so that it is just above the ground (inset). Begin a *Traveling Hip Twist* with your left hip by stepping forward with your left foot and twisting your left hip forward.

2 With your weight still on your right foot, twist your left hip back again. Try to keep your chest and upper body as still as you can, since this will help to make your hip movements look more dramatic.

At a glance

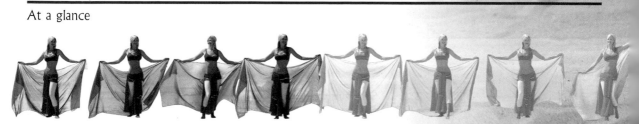

1 Step/Twist . . . . . 2 Twist . . . . . . 3 Step/Twist . . . 4 Twist . . . . . . 5 Hip Camel . . . 6 Hip Camel . . . . 7 Hip Camel . . . 8 Hip Camel

keep chest lifted

hands are relaxed but hold is firm

3 Perform a *Traveling Hip Twist* on the right side by stepping forward with your right foot and twisting your right hip forward.

4 With your weight still on your left foot, twist your right hip back.

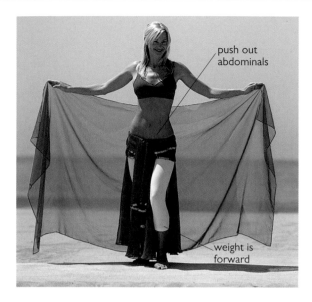

push out
abdominals

weight is
forward

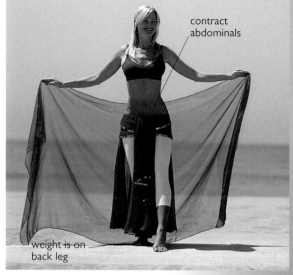

contract
abdominals

weight is on
back leg

5 Step forward with your left foot and perform the first half of a *Traveling Hip Camel* by bending your left knee and tilting your hips down.

6 Complete the *Traveling Hip Camel* by contracting your abdominals, straightening your left leg, and tilting your hips up. Keep your shoulders relaxed.

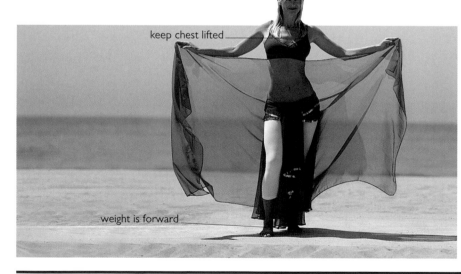

keep chest lifted

weight is forward

7 Step forward with your right foot and perform the first half of a *Traveling Hip Camel* by bending your right knee and tilting your hips down. Keep your arms in the same position, so that your veil flows behind you.

At a glance

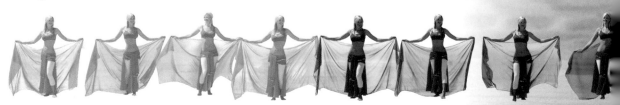

1 Step/Twist . . . . . . 2 Twist . . . . . . 3 Step/Twist . . . 4 Twist . . . . . . 5 Hip Camel . . . .6 Hip Camel . . . . 7 Hip Camel . . . . . 8 Hip C

keep shoulders relaxed

8 Finish the sequence by completing the *Traveling Hip Camel.* Contract your abdominals and tilt your hips up as you prepare to step forward with your left foot. As you do this, move your arms into *Classic Arms* with your left arm raised by your head.

VEIL DANCE, PART TWO

In this part of the dance you travel to the left, assuming three different arm positions over the eight counts. In the last four counts, notice how the undulations of the *Traveling Hip Snake* are complemented by the willowy movements of *Isis Arms*. As you lift your hip, raise your arm, and as you drop your hip, lower your arm.

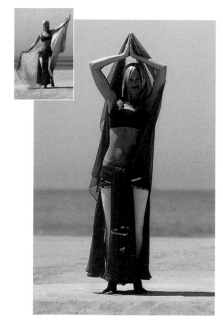

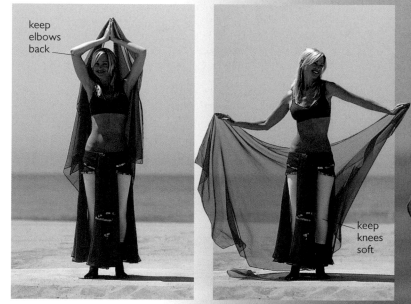

keep elbows back

keep knees soft

1 From the *Traveling Hip Camel* with *Classic Arms* (inset), step forward with your left foot so that your feet are parallel. Raise your hands above your head in *Temple Arms* and perform a *Head Slide* to the left.

2 With your arms in the same position, perform a *Head Slide* to the right. Be careful not to let your arms fall forward—they should frame your head movements.

3 Lower your arms and extend them just below shoulder level with elbows slightly bent. Begin to *Shoulder Shimmy*, keeping the movements small and rhythmic. Remember to keep your hips still.

At a glance

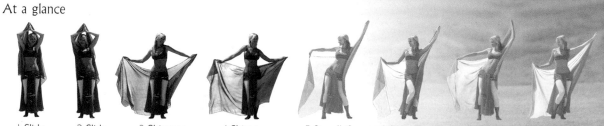

I Slide . . . . . 2 Slide . . . . . 3 Shimmy . . . . . . 4 Shimmy . . . . . . 5 Step/Lift . . . . 6 Slide/Drop . . . . 7 Step/Lift . . . 8 Slide/Drop

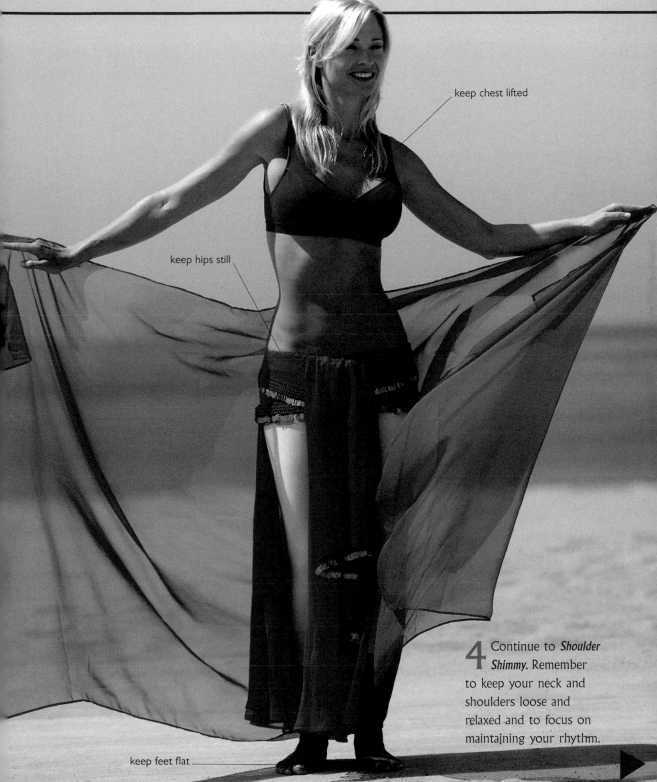

keep chest lifted

keep hips still

keep feet flat

4 Continue to *Shoulder Shimmy.* Remember to keep your neck and shoulders loose and relaxed and to focus on maintaining your rhythm.

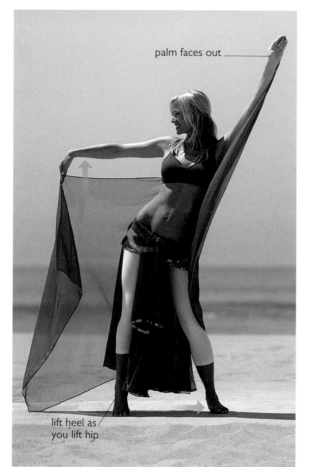

palm faces out

lift heel as
you lift hip

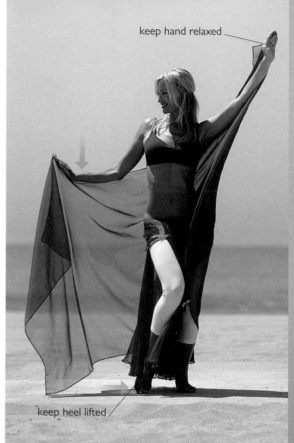

keep hand relaxed

keep heel lifted

5 Begin a *Traveling Hip Snake* to the left by stepping out to the side with your left foot and pushing out then smoothly lifting your right hip. As you do this, raise your left arm above your head and begin raising your right arm to perform *Isis Arms*. Your veil becomes almost like a wing.

6 Complete the *Traveling Hip Snake* by shifting your weight onto your left leg as you slide your right foot in to meet your left and drop your hip. As you do this, gracefully lower your right arm. Notice how your veil trails behind your arm, adding expression as you lower it.

At a glance

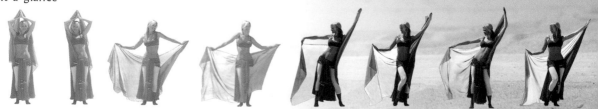

I Slide . . . . . 2 Slide . . . . . 3 Shimmy . . . . . . 4 Shimmy . . . . . . 5 Step/Lift . . . . 6 Slide/Drop . . . . 7 Step/Lift . . . 8 Slide/Drop

7 Perform another *Traveling Hip Snake*, traveling to the left by stepping out to the side with your left foot and pushing out then lifting your right hip. Raise your right arm as you continue to perform *Isis Arms*. As you do this, rotate your left hand inward so that your palm faces you.

palm faces in

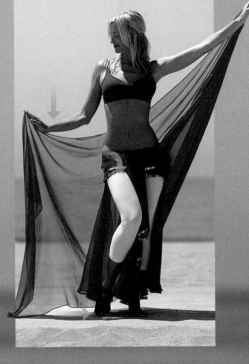

8 Complete the *Traveling Hip Snake* by shifting your weight onto your left leg as you slide your right foot in to meet your left and drop your hip. Finish the sequence by gracefully lowering your right arm as you complete *Isis Arms*. For dramatic effect at the end, flick your left hand so that your palm faces out.

VEIL DANCE FINALE

In this final dance sequence you move to your left, so when combined with Parts One and Two the entire dance forms an L-shape. Your feet start in a different position to the *Four–Count Turn* that you learned in the Basic Moves, but the footwork is the same. Use your veil for dramatic effect, and hold your head high like the fabulous goddess that you are.

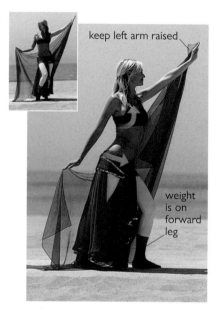

keep left arm raised

weight is on forward leg

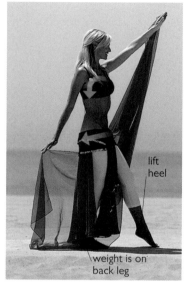

lift heel

weight is on back leg

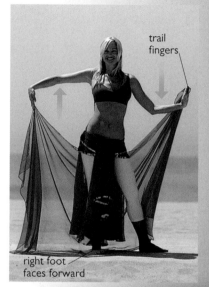

trail fingers

right foot faces forward

1 From the *Traveling Hip Snake* with left arm raised in *Isis Arms* (inset), turn to face left as you step back with your right foot and lower your right arm. Begin a *Body Wave*: Push forward and lift your chest, shift your weight forward, and tilt your hips down.

2 With your arms in the same position, complete the *Body Wave* by pulling your chest back and dropping it. As you do this, rock your weight back onto your right leg as you straighten your left leg and tilt your hips up.

3 Lower the heel of your left foot, and pivot on your right foot to turn and face forward. Simultaneously begin performing *Snake Arms* by gracefully raising your right arm as you lower your left arm.

At a glance

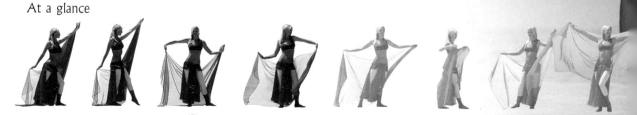

1 Body . . . . . . 2 Wave . . . . . 3 Snake Arms . . . 4 Snake Arms . . . . 5 Shift Forward . . . 6 Cross/Pivot . . . . 7 Step . . . . . . 8 Pose

keep hand relaxed
when holding veil

flick wrist up to add
movement to veil

4 Continue
performing
Snake Arms, raising
your left arm as you
gracefully lower your
right. As you do this, begin
shifting some of your weight
onto your left leg in preparation
for the *Four-Count Turn*.

left foot faces
direction of turn

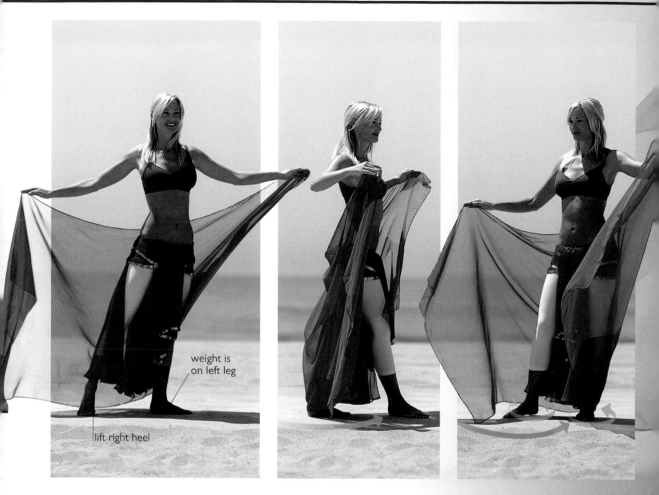

weight is
on left leg

lift right heel

5 Extend your arms at shoulder level at your sides with elbows soft as you begin a *Four–Count Turn* to the left by shifting your weight onto your left leg. Remember to keep your chest lifted and your shoulders level.

6 Step to your left, crossing your right leg in front of your left, and pivot around 180°. As you do this, begin bringing your hands together in front of you with fingertips facing.

7 Step around with your left foot and begin extending your arms at your sides. Move slowly and gracefully, allowing your veil to flutter behind you as you turn.

At a glance

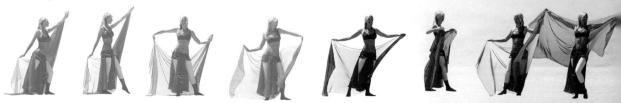

1 Body . . . . . . 2 Wave . . . . . 3 Snake Arms . . . 4 Snake Arms . . . . 5 Shift Forward . . . 6 Cross/Pivot . . . . 7 Step . . . . . . 8 Pose

bend left knee

weight is on
right leg

8 Complete the *Four–Count Turn* by stepping forward with your left foot, then shifting your weight onto your right leg. As you do this, strike your finishing pose— bend your left knee and raise your arms at your sides.

VEIL DANCE SUMMARY

Once you've learned the three eight-count parts of the Veil Dance, you'll find it easier to refer to this summary when performing the entire sequence. As before, moves on the right side are indicated with an "R" and moves on the left with an "L."

Veil Dance, Part One

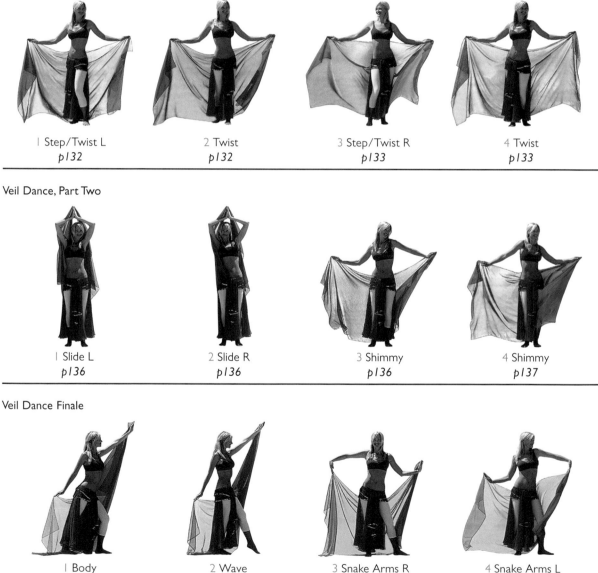

| 1 Step/Twist L | 2 Twist | 3 Step/Twist R | 4 Twist |
| *p132* | *p132* | *p133* | *p133* |

Veil Dance, Part Two

| 1 Slide L | 2 Slide R | 3 Shimmy | 4 Shimmy |
| *p136* | *p136* | *p136* | *p137* |

Veil Dance Finale

| 1 Body | 2 Wave | 3 Snake Arms R | 4 Snake Arms L |
| *p140* | *p140* | *p140* | *p141* |

Don't lose sight of the joy and the freedom that is intrinsic to bellydance.

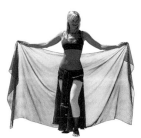

5 Hip Camel
p134

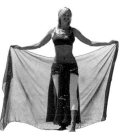

6 Hip Camel
p134

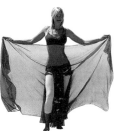

7 Hip Camel
p135

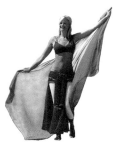

8 Hip Camel
p135

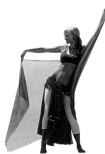

5 Step L/Lift R
p138

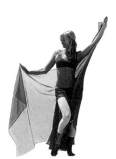

6 Slide R/Drop R
p138

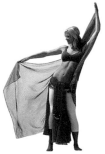

7 Step L/Lift R
p139

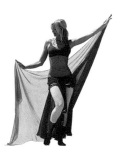

8 Slide R/Drop R
p139

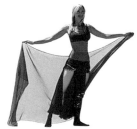

5 Shift Forward
p142

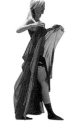

6 Cross/Pivot
p142

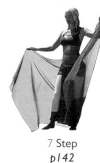

7 Step
p142

8 Pose
p143

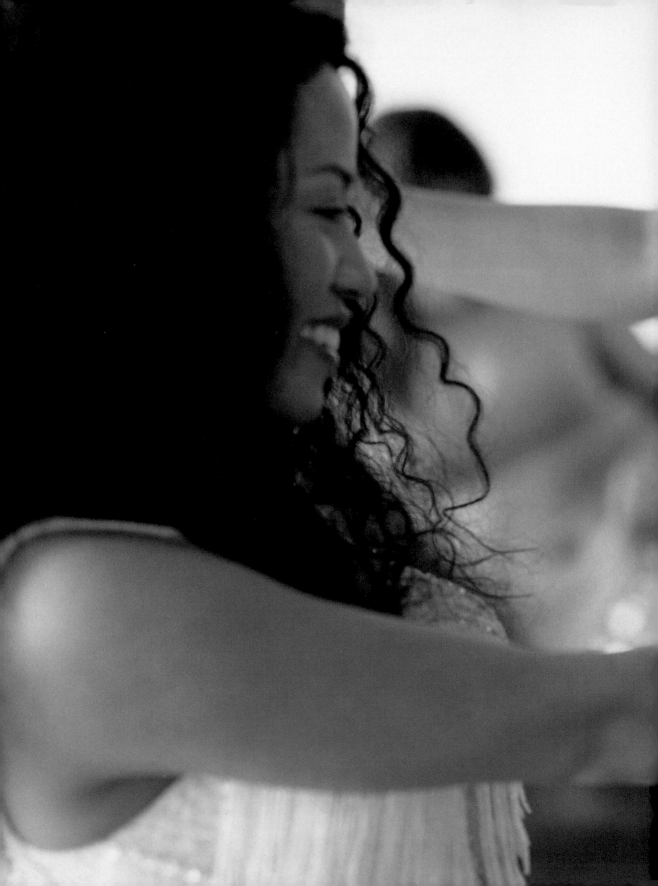

BELLY DANCE LIFESTYLE

You may have started bellydancing as a novel way to exercise but now find that you are intrigued by the colorful, flowing costumes or want to learn more about the traditional music to which you can dance. In the pages that follow I introduce you to the basics of costume as well as providing a brief introduction to Middle Eastern music, including recommendations to help you navigate your way through the many different styles. For those who want to share their dancing with others, I offer my advice, based on experience, for devising routines and performing them successfully.

COSTUME

A simple hip scarf or coin belt will help you to focus on your hips when you first begin bellydancing; and that may be the extent of your interest in costume. However, some students develop a true fascination with the colorful costumes of bellydance, and I for one believe that a gorgeous eye-catching outfit can enhance and intensify the dancing experience.

A professional bellydancer's costume is one of the tools of her trade. It must be beautiful as well as functional, since its purpose is to accentuate the bellydancer's movements. Costumes vary in design and decoration depending on the style of dance. For example, traditionally Turkish bellydancers perform more floorwork so they wear wide-legged harem pants rather than skirts.

The classic Cabaret-style costume shown opposite illustrates the standard components of a costume, which usually consists of four parts: Hip belt, bra, skirt, and arm accessories.

HIP BELT This fits snugly around the hips, leaving the belly free to perform Figure Eights and undulations. The belt can weigh up to about 8lb (4kg) and is made of stiff fabric to support the weight of the fringe and beads. The beads, in addition to being decorative, swing and glisten with the movement of the dancer and make subtle steps visible from a distance. Egyptian-style costumes have long beaded fringes, American Tribal ones are usually decorated with coins instead of the delicate beaded tassels shown opposite.

BRA Usually extremely ornate, the bra is reinforced to support the weight of the decorative coins, beads, or fringe. The design of the bra matches the belt. American Tribal dancers often wear a short, fitted top or vest known as a *choli* in addition to a bra; Turkish-style costume bras often drip with glittery sequins.

SKIRT In Cabaret-style bellydance, the dancer wears one or more circle skirts made of 6–10 yards (5.5–9m) of fabric that create a circle when the dancer spins. There are many other skirt designs that complement the style of dance performed. For instance, Egyptian dancers often wear the mermaid skirt which is form-fitting from the hips to the knee, then flares out. This style accommodates the delicate hip movements but allows for more complicated footwork since much of Egyptian-style bellydance is performed on the toes. Turkish bellydance involves more floorwork so harem pants (full-legged and gathered at the ankles) are often worn.

ARM ACCESSORIES These accentuate the dancer's graceful arm and hand movements. Gauntlets (fingerless gloves), armbands made of the same fabric as the costume, arm bracelets, or wrist cuffs may also be worn. Sometimes fabric is draped from the shoulder to the wrist and flows behind the arms as the dancer moves. Often the dancer holds a veil, which is made from 2½–3 yards (2.3–2.7m) of sheer fabric, such as chiffon, silk, nylon, or rayon, in a color that complements the costume. The veil can be ornamental or accentuate the dancer's elegant movements.

To say that collecting bellydance costumes is an expensive hobby is an understatement—a ready-made costume from Turkey or Egypt can easily cost over a thousand dollars. However, it is not difficult to assemble or even make a costume to fit your budget. Very basic and inexpensive costumes like the ones worn in dance routines two and three in this book consist of a pair of leggings and a simple bra top, a simple skirt—consisting of two panels of light-weight fabric that fall at the front and back—and a hip scarf. Of course, you can be as simple or as creative as you like—I have a costume made entirely of shells that I found on a beach.

Cabaret-style costumes are typically glamorous and ornately decorated. They help the bellydancer to feel feminine and confident.

epaulets made of strands of beads catch the light and jingle with movements such as the Shoulder Shimmy

beaded wrist cuffs accentuate delicate hand movements

decorative beading on the bra matches the hip belt

beaded tassels draw attention to the chest and belly

hip belt sits low on the hips and shows as much belly as possible

beaded fringe hangs from hip belt and jingles as the hips move

circle skirts are made of two contrasting colors of chiffon, which flows with the dancer's movements

slit in skirt allows for freedom of leg movements and provocatively exposes leg

beaded pharaonic panel draws attention to the legs and gives costume individual style

BELLYDANCE MUSIC

These pages are intended as a brief introduction to bellydance music, which is broadly categorized as Middle Eastern and includes many different styles. I have listed the names of some of the more popular musicians as well as making listening recommendations. You can then explore the music for yourself and decide what you like and what makes you feel like bellydancing.

MIDDLE EASTERN MUSIC

The complexities, overlapping rhythms, and intricate composition of Middle Eastern music make it sound incredibly exotic to the Western ear. When first listening and beginning to dance to it, try to identify the sounds of the different instruments (see *Middle Eastern Instruments*, opposite). The drums are the easiest to hear, since they generally provide the main rhythm, then let yourself be carried away by the heartfelt emotion that this music conveys. Love is a common theme in Middle Eastern music, so songs may sound melancholic but many are rhythmic and very exciting.

While Western music is based on a scale, or a key, Middle Eastern music is structured on a maqam. In Western music, the musical notes are a half-step (semi-tone) apart, with each of the 12 possible notes represented on the piano. Middle Eastern music has quartertones, pitches that are half-way between adjacent keys on a piano, so a maqam has twice as many notes as a Western scale. A maqam also tells the musician what the pauses are between notes and which notes are stressed.

In addition Middle Eastern music also has more complex rhythms with unusual time signatures. Where Western music might have an even-tempo 2/4 or 4/4 rhythm, Middle Eastern music may have a time signature such as 9/8, for example, which is common in Turkish music. See page 155 for information on where to buy Middle Eastern music, or for an introduction to it, try listening to www.radiobastet.com, an online radio station that plays vintage bellydance music.

DIFFERENT STYLES OF MUSIC

Most music stores have a Middle Eastern music section; this is where to begin looking for any of the different music styles and artists listed here.

CLASSIC CABARET Cabaret-style bellydancers perform to this music. You are most likely to hear it in restaurants and nightclubs. The songs are written specifically for bellydance and are very melodic with international influences and plenty of accents and rhythm changes to showcase the dancer's technical expertise.
Recommended listening: the Egyptian drummer, Hossam Ramzy, who has created many CDs specifically for bellydance, including: *Sabla Tolo* (great drum solos), *Baladi Plus Best of Oum Kalthoum, Best of Farid Altrash*; George Abdo; Setrak, a drummer who writes music specifically for bellydance; Jalilah, who produces music with Folk and Egyptian Orchestral influences.

EGYPTIAN ORCHESTRAL This emerged during the golden age of the Egyptian cinema, roughly between the 1930s and 1960s. During this time, a few extremely talented composers wrote many of the songs that remain popular today. Egyptian orchestral music is performed by professional musicians and contains many musical complexities not present in Folk music. This style of music embraced the large, 40-piece orchestra found in Western music and applied a uniquely Egyptian style to it.
Recommended listening: Mohamed Abdul Wahab, who wrote the classic songs "Zeina" and "Aziza;"

The composer and singer Farid al Atrash, whose most famous songs include: "Touta," "Zenouba," and "Ana Alli Wa Utilu;" Oum Kalthoum, an Egyptian national treasure, who made famous songs such as "Inte Omri," "Leilet Hob," and "Lisah Faker."

FOLK Middle Eastern folk music is played on traditional instruments crafted from available materials. The songs have a strong rhythmic pulse with simple melody lines that ordinary people with ordinary voices could sing. American Tribal style dancers dance to folk music. Its continuous rhythms make it ideal for novice bellydancers.

Recommended listening: Musicians of the Nile (Egyptian), Omar Faruk Tekbilek (Turkish), Orchestre National de Barbes (Algerian), Musicians of Jajouka (Moroccan).

FUSION This combines classic Middle Eastern music with another, usually Western, style of music.

Recommended listening: Alabina fuses Spanish and Arabic music; Chebbi Sabbah unites Indian and Arabic music with Electronica; Light Rain gives a Celtic flavour to Arabic music.

POP MUSIC *(Al Jeel)* This is the music currently heard on the radio and in nightclubs in the Middle East. The true rise of pop music began in the 1980s. Some of the music demonstrates a Western influence in the rhythms and instruments used.

Recommended listening: Pop music stars of Egypt are Amr Diam, Hakim, Warda, and Walid Tawfic. Tarkan is a Turkish pop singer; Cheb Khaled and Cheb Mami popularized *Rai*, Algerian pop music.

TURKISH This has similar rhythms to Egyptian music but uses more wind instruments such as the oboe and clarinet. It is characterized by the sounds of the *oud, ney, kanun,* and *dumbek.*

Recommended listening: Esin Engin is classic Turkish bellydance music; John Belizikjian is an extraordinary *oud* player. I highly recommend his CD *Gypsy Fire.*

MIDDLE EASTERN INSTRUMENTS

Familiarize yourself with the different instruments and the sounds that they make. When you dance, make each instrument correspond to a different type of movement or part of your body. The following is a list of the more popular Middle Eastern instruments:

DEF: This Egyptian instrument is a tambourine and frame drum in one. It is held by one hand while the other beats the rhythm.

DUMBEK: (Doom-behk) This hourglass-shaped drum provides the main rhythm of the band and is sometimes called a *darbouka.* Made of either clay or brass, it is played with the hand. It produces a flat vibrating "dum" sound and a sharper "tek" sound. Normally sharp, fast bellydance movements such as Hip Drops are performed to its beat.

KANUN: (Kah-NOON) A Turkish zither-like instrument, the *kanun* is like a harp but played horizontally on a table with moveable bridges. It has 72 strings that are played with pick-type rings placed on the tips of the index fingers. The *kanun* is a very ethereal sounding instrument, beautifully expressed with graceful arm movements.

NEY: This simple reed flute is about 2ft (90cm) long, with seven holes and no blowing tip. It produces a spiritual sound that is a perfect accompaniment to undulations and arm movements.

OUD: (ood) This 11-stringed Arabic instrument resembles a guitar but has a round body and a short neck. The *oud's* fingerboard does not have any frets, making it easier to improvise. It produces deep, soulful, haunting sounds perfect for Hip Shimmies, Figure Eights, and Hip Snakes.

ZILLS: This is the Turkish name for finger cymbals; in Arabic they are known as *sagat*. The small brass or silver disks are worn on the bellydancer's thumb and middle finger, a pair on each hand. They emit a high-pitched bell-like chime when struck together.

PARTIES AND PERFORMING

When you mention to friends that you are learning the ancient art of bellydancing, you are sure to get at least a raised eyebrow of interest—most people are intrigued by this mesmerizing dance. Now that you have mastered the Hip Snake and the shimmy, you may want to take it to the next level. You probably don't want to dance professionally, but you may have the urge to show your friends or your partner what you've learned with a performance.

Whether you are a professional or just showing your skills to your friends, your first performance can be unnerving. The following suggestions can be easily adapted for performing at a friend's baby shower, at a restaurant or bellydance party, or even in the bedroom.

PLANNING

One of the keys to success is good preparation. Here are advance planning tips for the novice performer:
• Aim to dance for between three and five minutes. This may not sound long, but time can feel as if it is going on forever when it is just you and your hips out there on the stage.
• Choose music that has a steady beat and that inspires you to dance. Prepare your music in advance—and make sure that it is the correct length for your routine.
• Find out how much space you will have for your stage (ideally, no less than 4x5ft [1x1.5m] and where your audience will be. Some dancers prefer to keep a little distance between them and their audience, others like more interaction and audience participation.
• Make an outline of your dance routine and practice it, but be prepared for the unexpected. Decide on two of your best bellydance moves; if you forget your routine or the unexpected happens, you can fall back on them.
• Choose a costume that makes you feel beautiful and that doesn't restrict your movements—it will distract you if you are worried about tripping up or fear that your costume might fall off (safety pin it where you can).
• Try to do a dress rehearsal before the performance.

CREATING ATMOSPHERE

If you are throwing a party, make the performance more memorable by decorating the room where you are going to bellydance.
• Place fragrant flowers or scented candles around the room. Scatter rose petals on the floor. Load your CD player with a varied selection of intoxicating and danceable bellydance music.
• Make the room where you are going to bellydance a Casbah by draping fabric and placing cushions on the floor along the walls. Rearrange furniture to allow enough room for your performance.

PERFORMING

Most importantly, assume a positive attitude before you begin. Remember that your audience want you to be good, and if you enjoy your performance, it's most likely that they will too.
• Put your music on before you begin (make sure it is audible!), and make a proud entrance, don't slink in.
• Be confident. Nothing is more attractive than confidence, and the best way to express it is to make eye contact and enjoy yourself.
• If nerves set in, pretend that you are dancing for yourself and that your audience is being treated to the pleasure of watching you. Perform your fall-back moves if you forget your routine.
• At the end of your show, hold your finishing pose and enjoy the applause, or take a gracious bow and disappear like a genie.

DEVISING YOUR OWN ROUTINE

Progressing from working through the basic moves to performing in front of an audience (even if it is made up of your friends) may feel like a big leap. I have provided routines in this book, but you may want to devise your own. Where do you begin?

You can use the routines in this book as starting points when devising your own dance sequences. Vary the order in which you perform the sequences, or edit them to suit your ability or taste. If there is a move that you feel less confident performing, replace it with another that is similar to it in style. For example, you can replace a sharp move like the Hip Lift with the Hip Pop, or a fluid move such as the Hip Snake with the Hip Camel.

You do not need a vast repertoire of different moves to create a good performance. It is much better to perform fewer moves well and with great energy and confidence than it is to exhaust yourself with an overly complicated routine.

Make your entrance and begin your routine with a song that is upbeat in tempo. An infectious song will not only catch your audience's attention, it can boost your confidence in your stage presence. I recommend starting with a traveling step where you walk toward your audience facing forward. Or, if you are surrounded, start by dancing a circle within the audience, creating a space for your stage in the midst of them. The tempo of the rest of the routine is up to you, but try to alternate between slow moves and faster, more spirited ones. If you begin to tire, dance more gentle, flowing moves such as the Figure Eight or Snake Arms while you recover. Finally, end with a dramatic pose and hold it to prompt the audience for applause— then stay there and enjoy it!

It's all about attitude!
Don't worry about what people are thinking; your delight in performing will be reflected in the faces of your audience.

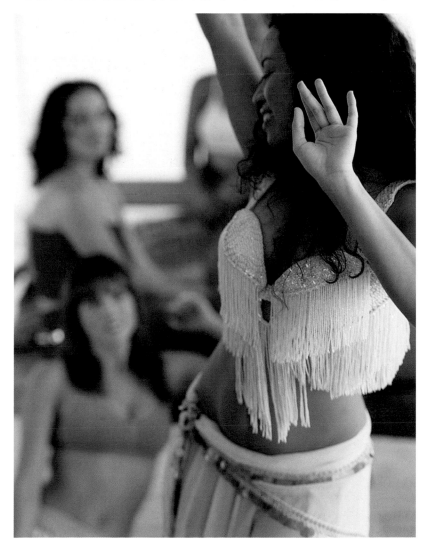

STYLES OF BELLYDANCE

Because bellydance has origins in many countries, several different styles have developed. Today, some dancers practice a particular style, but most borrow from many different styles to express themselves and make the dance their own. The following is a brief guide to some of the more popular styles of bellydance—it will help you to understand the origins of some of the moves that I teach in this book, but you can also use it as inspiration when creating your own dance style.

AMERICAN TRIBAL Although it borrows styles and costumes from many different historical periods and regions of the world (in particular India, North Africa, Afghanistan, and the Middle East), it is an American creation. Although still predominantly practiced in the US, it is beginning to spread further afield. Dancers perform in a troupe and dance with a unique cooperative method of spontaneous group choreography. Many dancers have body tattoos or facial drawings. They generally dance to Folk or world music.

CABARET Bellydancers who perform in restaurants and nightclubs in the West dance the Cabaret style. It is an amalgam of many different styles, including Turkish, Egyptian, and Folk. It is glamorous and exotic and this is reflected in the costumes, which are often ornately decorated. A Cabaret dancer may perform to Middle Eastern, Pop, Folk, or world music, or a combination of these. Cabaret dancers make a grand entrance, include dramatic moves in their routine, often dancing with a veil, and finish with a dramatic pose as demonstrated in the routines in this book. Although they borrow from many different styles of bellydance, a Cabaret-style dancer would never dance on her toes or perform floorwork.

FOLK AND ETHNIC This style is difficult to characterize. Different folk and ethnic styles are danced in different localized regions throughout the Middle East. In many areas styles have died out, so for this reason it is rare to find a dancer who can dance a faithful representation of a particular folk style. However, some moves can be traced back to particular folk styles, for example the Traveling Hip Twist belongs to the *ghawazee* style, an Egyptian folk-style of bellydance.

MODERN EGYPTIAN Also called Egyptian Cabaret, this is the contemporary Egyptian nightclub-style of bellydancing in which the dancer performs with a band that plays Egyptian Orchestral music. Much of the music that is danced to today was originally composed for movies made during the golden age of Egyptian cinema in the 1940s. In Egypt, it is common for a star dancer to perform with a 40-piece band. Outside of Egypt, a synthesizer usually duplicates the big band sound. The movements are refined and have obvious balletic influences with dancers performing tightly choreographed sequences, often dancing on the toes. In Modern Egyptian style, it is important to keep the upper body aligned over the hips. Costumes are customarily very glitzy and elaborately beaded, so it is not surprising that dancers generally don't perform floorwork.

TURKISH Highly improvisational, Turkish-style movements are "earthy" and incorporate backbends, floorwork (dancing with knees, hands, and back on the floor), and more pushing forward of the hips. A Turkish-style dance routine typically consists of five parts: an upbeat entrance while playing finger cymbals, or *zills*; a slower, more sensual sequence; a spirited, lively routine; a dance to a fast drum solo; and a playful, upbeat finale. The costumes are among the most risqué, baring plenty of leg and cleavage, and are often decorated with coins.

RESOURCES

Look out for bellydance classes at your gym, YWCA, or dance studios in your area. Or try any of the websites listed below, and they can put you in touch with local classes. Here, I also share some of my favorite stores and websites for buying music, costumes, and accessories. You might also consider going to a festival or even traveling to another country to see bellydancing or to shop—I provide some useful contacts for these options too.

FINDING A CLASS

www.shira.net
Directory of classes in the United States and around the world; nearly 800 listings.

www.zaghareet.com
Directory of classes throughout the United States.

www.bdancer.com
Directory of classes throughout the United States and abroad.

www.pinkgypsy.com
Directory of classes in Southern California.

www.bellydanceny.com
Directory of classes in New York.

www.helade.com
Directory of classes in New England.

BUYING MUSIC

www.amazon.com
Search this site using keywords: bellydance, Middle Eastern music, or enter the names of the musicians I mention on pages 150–151.

Arc Music
P.O. Box 111
East Grinstead, West Sussex
RH19 4FZ
Great Britain
www.arcmusic.co.uk
Good source for world music, and the music of Hossam Ramzy.

Artemis Imports
P.O. Box 68
Pacific Grove, CA 93950
Tel: (831) 373-6762
Fax: (831) 373-4113
www.artemisimports.com
Fantastic for bellydance music but also an excellent source for costumes and accessories; produce a mail-order catalog.

Pe-ko Records
5112 Hollywood Blvd,
Suite 108
Los Angeles, CA 90027
Tel: 323-664-8880
Fax: 323-664-1614
www.pekorecords.com
A Los Angeles-based music store; a good source for bellydance music of all styles.

Putumayo World Music
324 Lafayette St.
7th floor
New York, NY 10012
Tel: 212-460-0095
www.putumayo.com
Good selection of world music compilation CDs.

Rashid Music Sales Company
155 Court St.
Brooklyn, NY 11201
Tel: 1-800-843-9401
www.rashid.com
A New York-based music store; a good source for all styles of bellydance music. Excellent on-line selection of music.

www.dantzrecords.com
Website of John Bilezikjian, oud player.

www.dynrec.com/tekbilek
Website of Omar Faruk Tekbilek, the Turkish musician and singer.

www.hossamramzy.com
Website of Hossam Ramzy, a fantastic Egyptian drummer.

COSTUMES AND ACCESSORIES

www.bellydancerwear.com
Ready-to-wear Egyptian costumes and accessories.

Tribal Bazaar
517 Ocean Front Walk, #1
Venice Beach, CA 90291
www.tribalbazaar.com
Costume store selling tribal costumes and hip scarves with mail order available through their website.

Nature's Gems
1710 University Ave
Berkley, CA 94703
Tel: 510-548-2800
Fax: 510-540-1121
www.costlesscostumes.com
Website that specializes in costumes that are heavily decorated with coins.

Global Exchange
4401 Chadwick Rd.
Suite 702
Charlotte, NC 20211
Tel: 704-540-1460
Fax: 704-366-6042
www.thebellydanceshop.com
Ready-to-wear Turkish costumes and accessories.

Fatchancebellydance
P.O. Box 460594
San Francisco, CA 94146
Tel: 415-431-4322
www.fcbd.com
Website for San Francisco's American tribal bellydance troupe; they sell tribal costumes, accessories, and music through their mail-order catalog.

Saroyan Mastercrafts
P.O. Box 2056
Riverside, CA 92516
Tel: 909-783-2050
Fax: 909-276-8510
www.saroyanzils.com
Store and website selling finger cymbals.

www.ganeshabazaar.com
Website that sells hip scarves and skirts from India.

www.costumegoddess.com
Good website for buying patterns for making your own costumes.

BELLYDANCE MAGAZINES

Habibi
P.O. Box 42018
Eugene, OR 97404
www.habibimagazine.com
Tel: 541-688-2333
Fax: 541-688-9461
Oldest Middle Eastern dance publication and only one available on news-stands.

Jareeda
P.O.Box 680
Sutherline, OR 97479
www.jareeda.com
International Middle Eastern dance magazine.

Zaghareet!
P.O. Box 1809
Elizabeth City, NC 27906
www.zaghareet.com
Middle Eastern arts and culture magazine.

Rakas
P.O. Box 1768
Queanbeyan, NSW 2620
Australia
www.rakas.org
Middle Eastern dance and culture magazine.

The Gilded Serpent
www.gildedserpent.com
On-line Bellydance magazine.

FURTHER READING

Bentley, Toni, *Sisters of Salome*, Yale University Press, 2002
Explores the spread of the cultural phenomenon Salomania.

Carlton, Donna, *Looking for Little Egypt*, International Dance Discover Books, 1995
Biography of Little Egypt.

Devine Brown, Dawn, *Embellished Bras*, Ibexa Press, 2003
Guide to making your own bellydance costumes.

Skinner, Richard, *The Red Dancer*, Ecco, 2002
Biography of Mata Hari.

STUDY TOURS

Travel to another country to see bellydancing, shop, or take workshops.

www.casbahdance.org
Organizes study trips to Egypt to learn bellydance.

www.mesmera.com
Organizes study trips to Brazil and Africa to learn bellydance.

EVENTS/FESTIVALS

Cairo Carnival
A weekend in June with non-stop bellydance performances, classes, and shopping.
www.mecda.org

Rakkasah West
A weekend in March in San Francisco with bellydancing, shopping, and bellydance competitions.
www.rakkasah.com

Rakkasah East
A weekend in October in New York with bellydancers and vendors of costumes and accessories.
www.rakkasah.com

Kismet Dance Festival
A weekend bellydance festival in Utah in August.
www.kismetdance.com

Dolphina has produced a series of instructional DVDs and videos as well as CDs of bellydance music that make useful accompaniments to this book.

INSTRUCTIONAL DVDS AND VIDEOS

Introduction to Bellydance
An exhilarating 50-minute cardiovascular bellydance workout that increases flexibility while toning and contouring the body.

The Warrior Goddess—Beyond Basics
A 50-minute workout that shows you how to access, energize and isolate underdeveloped hip muscles.

Bellydance with Veils
A 30-minute workout incorporating veils that firms, sculpts, and strengthens the entire upper body.

Bellydance with Finger Cymbals
A 30-minute finger cymbal training routine which shows how to make your own music while enhancing your coordination and concentration and enriching your bellydance workout.

MUSIC CDS

The Introduction to Bellydance
Invigorating world percussion, sensual flutes, and healing ocean sounds.

The Warrior Goddess—Beyond Basics Bellydance
Lush melodies filled with powerful world percussion, sensual flutes, and exotic strings.

Bellydance with Veils
Dream-like melodies with ethereal flutes, strings, and percussion.

Bellydance with Finger Cymbals
Joyous melodies of dynamic world percussion and exotic grooves.

Spa Goddess
Subtle melodies infused with ocean sounds, soothing flutes, strings, and light percussion.

For further information, or to purchase DVDs, music, or costumes, contact: GoddessLife
Tel: 1-877-MYGODDESS
www.goddesslife.com

Dolphina teaches classes, organizes teacher training, and runs workshops at the Goddess Center.
Tel: 310-281-7447

INDEX

ACKNOWLEDGMENTS

AUTHOR'S ACKNOWLEDGMENTS

Without the following people, this fabulous book would not exist: A special thanks to everyone at DK for a gorgeous book, especially: Sharon Lucas and Tina Vaughan for having vision, Christopher Davis for putting my belly on the cover, Su St. Louis for being the Goddess at work (keep it light), Miesha Tate and Michelle Baxter for such pure beauty, and to my confidante, the exquisite Nasim Mawji, for the 1-hour cry, the wonderful parallel world at the Best Western, and for your undeniable brilliance, fierce talent, and irresistible charm.

Thanks to the entire Santa Monica survivor crew for enduring the heat and madness to make the most delicious photos: John Robbins for turning my difficult personal time into a vacation with dreamy photos; Troy Bass (it really does taste like Cotton Candy), Meike Selhausen (you can wash me with Evian anytime), and to my stunning models: Ava Carpentier, Clarissa Manansala, and Mahira.

Thanks to my classy agent, Alan Nevins; my chic publicist and friend, Dominic Friesen; my stylish sage, Pat Garling; my first editor, the fancy Kim Blish; my late-night writing cohorts, Ruby and Rex; my amazing teammate, Zach Leary, for radiating your love on me; Gary Lennon, for your support and for being my family; my creamsicle, Rocket Sapphire, for the inspiration; my cosmic twin, Marcella de la Luna, for reminding me of the magic; my Sisters, you'll always have my heart; Samara, my first bellydance teacher, for opening the door; my partner and biggest fan, Whitney Ransick, without whom this book would surely not exist; the dolphins, for saving my life; my students, for teaching me; bellydancers everywhere, for making the world a more feminine and beautiful place; and to the Goddess, without her grace I surely would not exist.

PUBLISHER'S ACKNOWLEDGMENTS

Dorling Kindersley would like to thank the photographer John Robbins and his assistants Troy Bass and Alex de Groot, Maike Selhausen for models' hair and make-up, and the models: Ava Carpentier, Dolphina, Clarissa Manansala, Mahira, Miesha Tate, and Amal Walton. Thanks to Bal Togs (www.baltogs.com) for kindly supplying models' clothing and to Marika (www.marika.com) for supplying clothing from the Shiva Shakti Collection. Thanks also to Jennifer Williams, Stephanie Farrow, and Shannon Beatty for editorial assistance, Ros Saunders for design assistance, Miranda Harvey for creative design input, Nanette Cardon for the index, and Chrissy McIntyre for picture research and arranging the loan of clothing.

PICTURE CREDITS

The publisher would like to thank the following for their kind permission to reproduce their photographs:
(Abbreviations key: t=top, b=bottom, r=right, l=left, c=center)
8: Dave King; 9tl: The New York Public Library/Art Resource, NY; 9br:Bettmann/Corbis.

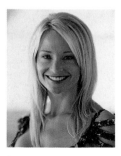

ABOUT THE AUTHOR

Dolphina began bellydancing at the age of four and later trained at the American Academy of Dance and Drama in New York City. She is a fitness instructor, certified by the American Association of Fitness, a Sivananda-certified yoga instructor, and a professional bellydancer. She has fused the best elements from her fields of expertise to create a unique exercise regime known as the Goddess Workout which she has taught at Crunch gyms across America. She produced her own Goddess Workout videos and DVDs, and owns her own studio in Los Angeles, California, where she runs classes and teaches women from all walks of life, from mere mortals to A-list celebrities. Her television credits include *Sex in the City*, *Live with Regis*, *Access Hollywood*, CNN, and *Lifetime*. She has been featured in numerous newspapers and magazines, including *Time*, *Glamour*, *Cosmopolitan*, *Self*, *US*, and *Fitness*. She founded her company, GoddessLife, in 1999 based on her philosophy that every woman is a Goddess.